PELICAN BOOKS

YOGA & MEDICINE

Steven F. Brena was born in Italy in 1921 and received his medical education and training in Italy, France, England, and the United States. For many years he has studied Yoga and Hindu philosophy in connection with problems of mental and physical hygiene. In addition to *Yoga & Medicine,* publications to his credit include *Bandengebiet* (a World War II novel published in Italian in 1947), numerous clinical and research writings, and *Pain and Religion: A Psychophysiological Study.* Dr. Brena was formerly an Assistant Professor of Anesthesiology at the University of Washington Medical School. He is currently on the staff of St. Joseph Hospital in Lewistown, Idaho.

STEVEN F. BRENA, M.D.

Yoga & Medicine

The Merging of Yogic Concepts
with Modern Medical Knowledge

Edited by Silvio G. Brena

Penguin Books

Penguin Books
625 Madison Avenue
New York, New York 10022

Penguin Books Canada Limited
41 Steelcase Road West
Markham, Ontario, Canada L3R 1B4

First published by The Julian Press, Inc., New York, 1972
Published in Pelican Books 1973
Reprinted 1975, 1976

Printed in the United States of America by
Kingsport Press, Inc., Kingsport, Tennessee

. . . Together,
for a quarter of a century,
we have been seeking for the Truth;
together we came to rest among free
men, on the Altar of inner Peace:
to my Wife.

... "Remaining immersed in Yoga, perform all
actions forsaking attachment to their
fruits. Remain indifferent to success and
failures while performing all actions.
The mental evenness during all states of
activities resulting in success or failure
is termed YOGA."

The Bhagavad Gita II:48

... "Pure spiritual life is the inverse resolution
of the potencies of Nature, which have emptied
themselves for the Whole Man. Or it is the
return of the power of pure Consciousness to
its essential form (Cosmic Consciousness)."

The Yoga-Sutra of Patanjali, 4:34.

Contents

Diagrams and Figures

Preface

This book has been written for the general public. In order to make it more enjoyable, I have often used dramatized and imaginative language to express physiological concepts, with many examples drawn from everyday, habitual experiences.

There are many ways to present the same idea; in using words borrowed sometimes from medicine, sometimes from philosophy and religion, often from common sense, I hope I have kept open communications with the reader.

To the health professionals I apologize if they find some concepts in this book an oversimplification of theories and models still controversial and far from being fully understood, such as the "spinal gate theory," present-day thinking about nutrition, pulmonary physiology, and so on. An academic and detailed discussion of controversial issues would have been pointless in a book designed for the general public. By the same token, since I am not a professional Orientalist and philosopher, I am sure that some expert in these fields of knowledge will find few of my ideas not really orthodox and not completely in agreement with current theories.

I am, however, confident that all of them will understand that this book is not intended to discuss difficult and controversial issues, but simply to challenge some plain thinking in connection with very common human problems of health, diseases, physical, and mental hygiene.

Steven F. Brena

February, 1972
Mercer Island, Washington

Introduction

To discuss "Yoga" among Western cultures is rather difficult, as this term has been given so many misinterpretations ranking from mistaking Yoga for "occultism," hypnotism, and "spiritualism," to labeling it a simple physical training, along with the misled idea that it gives extraordinary powers to the person undertaking it.

Since I intend to discuss Yoga using a language borrowed from medicine, I deem it necessary, from the beginning, to identify the ground upon which I shall move, in advance apologizing to those readers who are acquainted with the topic, if they find repeated in this introduction concepts and definitions they already know from well-qualified books on Yoga.

The testimony of great saints and sages in all ages teaches that man is a soul expressed in a body through the working of the mind. It also says that man is often unaware of his spiritual nature, turned as he is toward a pre-eminent body identification. In this basic mistake, most of our human disharmonies find their origin.

YO-GA is a Sanskrit word meaning "Re-Union"; the same root can be found in the Latin *con-jungo*, in the French *conjoindre*, in the English *to join*. In the actual Hindu meaning,

the term "Yoga" stands first for the correction of the human
disharmonies into a harmonious unity, then for the reunion of
the human entity with God, within and above the creation.
Let me remark here that a similar concept can be traced back
to the word *Religion,* derived from the Latin *re-ligo*—to join,
to bind together.

The philosophical system called *Yoga,* one of the three great
systems of the Hindu Philosophy (1, 2, 29), claims a divine
origin in the teaching that Lord-Krishna gives to his disciple
Arjuna on the battle field of Hastinapûra, according to the
Bhagavad-Gita, the *Song Celestial* of Hinduism. In the *Gita,*
Krishna is often referred to as *Yogiswara*—Master of Yoga (17
6, 29).

Historically, the Yoga philosophy seems to date back several
centuries B.C., and it is believed to have been codified by the
Hindu philosopher Patanjali, whose *Aphorisms,* known as
Yoga-Sutras, are now well known in the United States through
excellent English translations (19-29).

In reality, Yoga is but a slow, deep, intelligent, re-elaboration
of a very old body of knowledge, transmitted from generation
to generation through the teaching of enlightened masters, the
so-called *rishis.* They were the sages and the poets of a splendid
Hindu civilization that flourished in India about one thousand
years B.C., and expressed through the *Vedas,* the oldest sacred
scriptures in all the history of mankind.

The Yoga system includes several "paths" or "ways" through
which the same goal—the glorification of God in man—is
sought. *Jnāna* Yoga—the "Yoga of knowledge"—teaches how
to achieve the goal through wisdom, understanding, and
knowledge, obtained from "Right Thinking," that is, from the
exercise of "Practical Reason"—to use a term borrowed from
the German philosopher E. Kant (17, 18, 19, 20). *Karma* Yoga
—the "Yoga of action"—adopts "Right Living" as the means
to spiritual perfection. By "Right Living" the Hindu philosophers mean the mystique of work and duty in their pure forms,
devoid of all egotistical desires for material profit. The first
lesson delivered by the Lord-Krishna to his disciple Arjuna, in
the imminence of the battle, is a lesson of *Karma* Yoga (25).
Gandhi is, no doubt, the greatest *Karma* Yogi of modern India
(9, 10, 26). The Christian equivalent of "Right Living" can be

easily found in the practical exercise of charity and service to our fellow men.

Bhakti Yoga—the "Yoga of devotion"—emphasizes the role of love as the way to attain God-communion. Devotional practices, rites of worship, devotional chanting, inspiring religious *Satsangas* (devotional meetings), are prevalent on this Yogic path. In the history of Christian mysticism, St. Francis of Assisi probably is one of the most perfect examples of an enlightened *Bhakti* Yogi, as shown by the infinite love toward all aspects of creation that he manifested in his teachings.

Haṭha Yoga—the "Yoga of health"—seeks primarily to correct our physical and mental disharmonies through a balanced program of bodily and mental training. Probably, it is the best known form of Yoga in the Western world, popularized by a rich bibliography and partially re-elaborated in many exercises of contemporary physical education (14, 15, 16).

Finally, *Raja* Yoga—the "Yoga of self-realization"—the Royal Yoga, is so defined because it epitomizes all the forms of Yoga (thought, action, and devotion) into a perfect synthesis, adding precise techniques of superior psychophysical training. It is considered the highest form of Yoga, the closest to Patanjali's original teachings. To Raja Yoga rightfully belongs the evocative definition "Path on the Razor's Edge," which can be traced back to the *Upanishad,* pointing out the difficult ascent of man toward God (22, 23).

A modern form of *Rāja* Yoga, particularly suited to Western people, was worked out between the end of the nineteenth and the beginning of the twentieth century by three great Yogis of modern India, Babaij, Lahiri Mahasaya, and Sri Yuktesvar, who passed it on to the West through one of their greatest disciples, Paramahansa Yogananda, founder of an American Institute of Yoga Studies and Teachings, the "Self-Realization Fellowship," with legal seat in Los Angeles, California (26, 27, 28, 30, 32).

Although it claims a divine origin, and teaches how to achieve a mystical God-communion, Yoga is not an organized religious denomination. Rather it offers excellent support to all formal religious doctrines. It ultimately exalts the individual adhesion to our fathers' faith, setting up spiritual examples for the community of the faithful.

In this book, I propose to discuss some of the human phenomena as they are currently viewed in contemporary medicine, and will attempt to demonstrate connections, similarities,
sometimes identities, between Yogic ideas and medical concepts. It is my hope that this might help to correct some biases,
misinterpretations, and wrong judgments about this venerable
expression of an ancient and enlightened civilization, which
has outlived time and has risen above historical vicissitudes.

Learning of the medical basis for benefits obtainable through
the practice of Hatha Yoga, perhaps some readers will be
tempted to make some further investigation on the subject,
looking for serious references in order to obtain practical
instructions. A few others, hopefully, will be willing to start
the first steps toward the joyous summits of *karma, bhakti,* and
Rāja Yoga, standing up as living examples of faith and hope
in the human condition.

I am providing at the end of this text a list of references on
Yoga and related topics, which I have consulted before writing
the present book. The numbers in parentheses refer to quota-
tions drawn from the references.

Part One

Some
Biological
Functions
in Humans:
The Yoga
Point of View

Chapter One

The Integral Man:
A View of
Our Nervous
System

We could look at our body as a highly sophisticated machine in which two great systems can be distinguished: an outer system and an inner system. Through the former, man is connected and interrelates with the external world, which is his outer environment; we can call this organization a "somatic system" or a "system of relation." The inner system, on the other hand, provides for the vital functions and maintains and sustains our life; we can call it the "vegetative" or "visceral system." Through this delicate visceral organization, man keeps his "inner environment" balanced, this expression meaning a good functioning of the sets of cells and tissues that make up the human body.

The Somatic System

The somatic system of relation is formed by the sense organs: sight, hearing, taste, touch, smell, and by the organs of motion: muscles, bones, and articulations. The operation of the sense and the motion organs is controlled by a "power plant" situated in various well-defined areas of the brain. From the "motor" areas, an intricate network of nerve fibers originates, like the numerous wires of a very complex electrical machine, down they go along the vertebral spine, forming, like a cord, the so-called "spinal cord." At various levels of the vertebral spine, nerve fibers emerge from the cord, forming the well-known peripheral motor nerves. These nerve trunks go to the muscles of the body, in the head, in the neck, in the trunk, and in the four limbs, carrying to them the electrical impulses generated by the brain's "electrical power." Schematically, the function of the muscle is dependent upon three different factors: a trigger mechanism in the brain (volitional or conditioned), an electrical impulse, a contraction under the electrical discharge. Three forms of energy are, therefore, required for any voluntary muscular contraction: a volitional energy, an electrical energy, an elastic energy (stored in the muscle). Actually, these different forms of energy are nothing else but bioelectrical transformations of one and the same vital energy of which modern science does not know very much as far as its inner source is concerned.

From the muscles, the bones, the sense organs, from every square millimeter of skin, over the entire surface of the body, other numerous nerve fibers originate; they cluster successively in nerve trunks, called peripheral sensory nerves. They enter the spinal cord at various levels of the vertebral spine, where they climb up toward the sensorial areas of the brain. Over the sensory nerves, information about various sensations, such as cold, warm, pain, touch and pressure, is transmitted to the brain's "power plant." Some very sensitive brain centers are located in those areas called brain stem and medulla oblongata, where information concerning vital functions correlated with life phenomena is received and elaborated upon. Schematically, a sensation, like the muscular contraction, is made up of three different components: a sensory stimulus (a light, a sound, a pin-prick), an electrical impulse over sensory nerves, and an "electrical bell" in the brain, activated upon the arrival of the sensory impulse. The "electrical bell" in turn triggers a number of mental interpretative functions, which will be briefly discussed in the next chapter. An intricate system of electrical relays sets the sensory brain centers into electrical circuits with the motor centers, so that proper muscular activity can be started following the "ringing of the bell" and its interpretation. The bell ringing upon sensory reception may reach the level of conscious cognition, consequently triggering a voluntary movement; or it may just "ring" at some semi-conscious or unconscious level, generating automatic and reflex muscular activity (such as the retraction of one's hand when it comes into contact with a hot object). Voluntary muscular actions are relatively few compared to automatic and reflex movements. The blinking of the eyelids following light flashes, the knee-jerks and all other jerks, the turning of the head toward the source of a sound, are all examples of reflex and automatic activities upon the reception of a sensory impulse.

The Vegetative System

The vegetative system is composed of two sections: the para-sympathetic and the sympathetic system. Each includes centers of nervous tissue, called ganglia, and a dense network of small nervous fibers running from the ganglia to all the vital organs of the body, regulating their respective functions. The ganglia are joined together by a rich network of intercommunicating nerve fibrils, forming altogether a few vegetative nerve plexuses.

Human anatomy distinguishes five nerve plexuses: (1) the cranial plexus (parasympathetic), containing fibers of vital importance to life (the so-called vagus nerve); among many functions, it governs the activities of the heart, the lungs, the stomach, and part of the intestines; (2) the cervicothoracic plexus (sympathetic), located at the base of the neck, with nerve fibers going to the heart and to the lungs and to the blood vessels in the upper limbs and in the face; (3) the thoracolumbar plexus (sympathetic), at the level of the lower thoracic and first lumbar vertebra, otherwise called *coeliac plexus* or *solar plexus,* with fibers to the stomach, the liver, the spleen, and the upper part of the intestines; (4) the lumbar plexus (sympathetic), at the level of the lower lumbar verte-brae, with fibers to the kidneys, bladder, uterus (in the female), and to the blood vessels in the lower limbs; (5) the sacrococcy-geal plexus (parasympathetic), at the level of the sacrum. The regulation of the sexual functions depends mainly on the sacral plexus.*

---

* Most likely the original etymology of the word *sacrum* for this bone may be found in its connection with the nervous system attending to the sexual activity, the importance of which as the giver of life was stressed by primitive religious rites.

The sympathetic and the parasympathetic vegetative activities are quite different in physiological character. Roughly, the sympathetic can be viewed as a "positive" force stirring up vital functions and activating hormonal secretions, whereas the parasympathetic can be considered a "negative" force, quieting down vital functions and providing for their basic needs. For example, under sympathetic predominance, heartbeats are accelerated and the blood pressure goes up, whereas when the parasympathetic takes over, the heart rate and the blood pressure slow down.

A healthy functioning of the human body, therefore, is heavily dependent upon a harmonious correlation between the two sections of the vegetative system in their effects upon each one of our visceral organs and blood vessels. In the average humans, as in the animals, both the sympathetic and the parasympathetic activities are totally autonomous, removed from any conscious control of the individual will power.

The whole vegetative nervous system is joined in a close functional connection to two areas of the brain not controlled by one's subjective consciousness, called *thalamus* and *hypothalamus*. From these areas and from centers of nervous substance similar to the vegetative ganglia (the so-called lymbic system), nerve fibers diverge in great quantities either down the sympathetic and parasympathetic plexuses, or up to the conscious cerebral cortex. The thalamus and hypothalamus therefore constitute a sixth center of the vegetative nervous system, situated in the brain.

The vegetative system functions in ways quite different from those of the somatic system. To form an approximate idea of its operation, one must picture the vegetative system in man as a perfect room thermostat. Just as a room thermostat intervenes automatically to control the surrounding temperature when the latter departs from its prefixed limits, so the sympathetic and parasympathetic nervous plexuses intervene, automatically and in a way totally removed from one's conscious will, to regulate the proper operation of the internal organs essential to life. The role of the brain centers in the above-mentioned regulating mechanism is not quite clear. It is likely that the thalamus and the hypothalamus function as a sort of

radar capable of warning the vegetative nervous plexuses imme-
diately, in case something goes wrong anywhere in the organs.

However utterly different in their anatomic structure and
functional meaning, the somatic system of relation and the
vegetative system are strictly connected to each other. This
connection is anatomically formed by a thick network of connecting nerve fibers running through vegetative ganglia and
motor and sensory nerve trunks along their entire course in
the vertebral column, in the brain stem, in the areas of the
thalamus and of the hypothalamus, up to the conscious cerebral cortex. Through these innumerable relays (to use a term
well known in electrical technology), the vegetative plexuses
are set into circuit with the somatic system, so that the bioelectrical impulses traveling on the two great nervous networks affect one another in turn.

To continue our electrotechnical comparison, we can imagine the whole nervous organization of man as a huge and very
complex electrical system, conceived so that by switching on a
light in any one of its points, a flux of current is simultane-
ously felt in all the other points of the system, a flux more or
less intense, more or less capable of switching on other lights
indirectly, nonetheless always noticeable to the recording of a
galvanometer. This statement is literally true, as the recording
of electrical currents in the heart, in the brain, and in the
muscles, amply demonstrates. The average man has only a partial voluntary control of his electrical system, so that he is only
capable of switching on a few lights at will. He cannot send
voluntary electrical energy over all the circuits of the entire
system. In fact, he is capable of contracting and relaxing his
back and limb muscles, but he absolutely cannot control the
rhythm of his heart or command his stomach and liver.

I have compared the nervous impulses to an electrical current. Actually, the intimate mechanism of nervous conduction is
a bit more complicated than a simple electrical current. A nervous impulse has rather the character of a bioelectrochemical
phenomenon through the presence of certain particular chemical substances, like adrenalin and acetylcholin, forming at the
end of the nerve fibers because of the impulse itself. We can
think of the nervous impulse as a wave of electrochemical

energy, with positive and negative polarity, which goes through the nerve and condenses into a microscopic drop of adrenalin or acetylcholin. Through a biochemical process, this drop in turn causes the contraction of the muscle or the motion of the organ it comes into contact with.

In the government of human life, both vegetative and somatic, still a third powerful and complex factor intervenes. I mean the endocrine glands, which everybody has certainly heard of. There are eight main endocrine glands in man— hypophysis, thyroid, thymus, suprarenal (bilateral), pancreas, and sex glands (bilateral). The endocrine glands are in close functional connection with the nervous system. In fact, nerve fibers leave the sympathetic and parasympathetic ganglia and head for the endocrine glands, setting them into circuit with the vegetative system and hence, indirectly, with the system of relation.

Each endocrine gland produces one or more hormones. Each hormone exercises multiple actions of regulation over vital phenomena, whose detailed analysis lies beyond the subject matter of this book. For our purposes, it matters to note here that in their intimate essence the hormones are but further manifestations of electrochemical energy condensed in very small quantities inside the cells and tissues of the human body. An example of this is provided by adrenalin, a substance either formed by the suprarenal glands as a hormone, or condensed at the end of the sympathetic nerve fibers because of the bio-electric impulse.

As in the case of his vegetative nervous system, man also has poor control over his hormones, being mostly dominated by them. The phrase so many times relevantly and irrelevantly repeated, "man is the product of his endocrine glands," is true for the average person. It is enough to think of the painful irritability and emotional frailty of those persons with an over-active thyroid—the so-called hyperthyroid people—or of the sexual problems that often mark a dysfunction of the sex glands.

To summarize this intricate, though brief, attempt to describe human anatomy and nervous physiology, we can sketch the whole matter figuratively as follows: In that individual entity, called man, actually "three men" coexist, distinct one from the other. One man we can define as "somatic man." This man is conscious of himself, and lives in the external world, which he communicates with voluntarily through his system of relation—cortical areas of the brain, motor and sensory nerves, muscles, sense organs. The modalities of operation of this somatic man, as they evolve with reference to his environment, to the education received, to the experiences lived, constitute the so-called personality (from the Latin *persona*—"mask"), with its defects and its virtues, its passions and its aspirations, its habits and its relative automatisms.

A second man, not normally conscious of himself, we can call "vegetative man." This man does not communicate with the external world, and therefore, does not appear to the eyes of the world, but his role is so important that the whole individual personality is influenced by him—thalamus, hypothalamus, vegetative plexuses, nervous relays with the spinal cord. The vegetative man silently works to maintain his mundane, somatic brother, in equilibrium with his internal surroundings, that is, to make sure that the internal organs indispensable to life work to perfection. The external world can affect him through the neurovegetative and spinal relays and damage his functional perfection. Often his worst enemy is his very individual brother, the somatic man, who in order to indulge in somatic passions, demands unusual efforts of him.

As long as the vegetative man can satisfy the whims and the intemperances of his somatic brother, the individual personality can appear firm and harmonious. But when the equilibrium breaks, the personality too breaks, and numerous disabilities appear. Often the vegetative man takes vengeance for his brother's intemperance, and tortures him underhandedly, even though the latter would like to stay quiet, imposing on him the law of his primeval instincts and of the habits learned during his past experiences. A habit could be figuratively defined as follows: when the somatic man repeatedly teaches the vegetative man some behavior, the latter learns the lesson and plays it back again and again, even against the will and the interest of the somatic brother who yet had been the cause of it. For instance, if your stomach learns to like alcohol, it will keep asking for it, even if you would like to stop drinking.

Between the somatic man and the vegetative man, not always in a friendly relationship, is included the third man, whom we can call "hormone man"—unconscious areas of the brain, endocrine glands, neurovegetative relays. The hormone man is only vaguely aware of himself, mostly in the sexual sphere, and collaborates preferably with the vegetative man whom he often protects against his somatic brother's intemperances by depriving the latter of the hormonic contribution he needs to keep going. Typical is the case of premature sexual exhaustion in individuals obsessed by sex.

The three parts of man, the three functional "men," are bound together to form an entity indivisible by that bioelectrical fluid called nervous, or "vital" energy, omnipresent in every particle of the human body, whose functional expression condenses into acetylcholin, adrenalin, and hormone substances.

Three men in one: a human trinity analogous but not similar to the Divine Trinity. For, even though in the human trinity one is the substance, distinct in three parts, three ways of being, yet each of the parts lacks the harmony with the whole, consequently lacks the "One" which the three parts constitute, the attribute of spiritual perfection.

At this point, allow me a brief annotation of a theological nature, to make us reflect on the agreement between our contemporary knowledge and Biblical teaching. The latter shows man as a being impoverished of his primitive divine spiritual perfection through the sin of Adam and Eve. The former confirms, on the human level, the imperfection of the average man who is unaware of his wholeness and consequently does not have integral control over himself. Those individuals we designate by the name of Men, those Men we address by the pronoun "you," or whom we think of by the pronoun "I," in their greater part are Men only by a third, the other two thirds being quite unconscious of their humanity. The spiritual and material consequences of this human disharmony are dramatic, and are whispered by countless individuals in the privacy of the confessional or of a doctor's office.

To bring oneself back again to one's totality, recovering the conscious control of one's three parts, to fuse the three men into One Man, re-establishing the ontological harmony and order—this is the higher task of human behaviors, entrusted to man during his lifetime, his real reason of being, distinct from the animal world. Yoga is an efficacious method, millenary in experience, to reach this noble goal more rapidly and more securely.

So we come to the discussion of Yoga. First let us examine in a little more detail its neurological analogies with modern medical knowledge, keeping in mind that what will be discussed here must be considered as an analogy of thought and of functional hypothesis rather than as a real anatomic and physiological identity. In fact, the Hindu science was not acquainted with the art of sectioning human corpses anatomically. Its knowledge of man is the sole result of an intelligent and minute observation of the vital phenomena, backed by a unitarian conception of the entire universe of which man is but a miniature.

Center of gravity and of energy irradiation, according to Yoga teachings, is the cerebrospinal axis formed by the brain contained in the skull, and by the spinal cord which is enclosed in the column formed by the vertebrae. Along this cerebrospinal axis there are five functional spinal centers plus a sixth center situated inside the skull, whose projection can be located on one's forehead at a point resting exactly between the two eyebrows (the Hindus call this point "center of superconsciousness").* The functional centers of the Yoga physiology are called *Chakras* in Sanskrit, and roughly correspond to the vegetative nervous plexuses, such as they have been revealed by anatomic dissection.

Modern Yoga teaching, in an effort to make comprehension simpler for us Westerners, is inclined to forget the ancient Sanskrit name of each *Chakra,* and assume names analogous to medical words. As a matter of fact, it talks about an upper medullar center and five spinal centers: cervical, thoracic, lumbar, sacral, and coccygeal. But similar names must not arouse confusion of concept. I want to insist on the fact that the

---

* If you are familiar with archaeological museums, you will have noticed that almost all the artistic representations of human figures, from ancient Oriental civilizations, have their eyes turned upward, almost as if they were concentrated on their foreheads.

Chakra does not have an anatomical structure like its homonymous sympathetic or parasympathetic plexus, being a purely functional unit, a center capable of picking up and distributing vital energy, as we shall examine in more detail later on. Anatomic entity or center of energy, the fundamental concept common to Yoga and medicine remains, however, identical. Each *Chakra,* like its equivalent vegetative plexus, controls the function of one or more internal organs. For example, the work of the heart is controlled by a *Chakra* called *Anāhata,* whose medical equivalent is the cervicothoracic plexus. Further, the sexual function is placed under the control of the *Mūlādhāra Chakra,* or sacrococcygeal plexus.

In the Yoga conception, each *Chakra* has a double polarity whose Sanskrit name, *pingala+iḍa,* could be freely translated as "positive pole" and "negative pole." Therefore, the five spinal *Chakras* and the sixth upper endocranial *Chakra* constitute altogether twelve centers of energy irradiation (6 positive+6 negative), which form a system the Yoga Doctrine calls "astral," comparing the *Chakras* to the constellations of the Zodiac. This "astral system," hidden along man's vertebral column, constitutes sort of a "second man" inside the material covering of the physical body, in close relationship with the inner environment. So, also in the Yoga terminology, the concept of human entity appears distinct in two parts: the "carnal" or "material" man corresponds to our somatic man, whereas the "astral man" roughly corresponds to our vegetative man.

The Yoga doctrine also considers a "third man" who is, however, completely different from my definition of the "hormone man." It is called the "Spiritual or Ideal Man," and it is identifiable as pure spirit, divine image buried in the human consciousness, ontological presence of God within us. The Western concept of the "Soul" is close to the Hindu conception of the "Ideal Man."

Yoga, too, recognizes the separation of the different parts of the human entity, and the fact that human consciousness is mostly limited to the material body. The entire Yoga training is a well-coordinated effort to bring together the material and the astral man into a harmonious functioning, then to awaken the Spiritual Man within, so to complete a perfect unity in trinity.

But here I have drifted into a religious discussion, and consequently I am treading a field not pertaining to the specific purpose of this book. Instead, I invite those readers who are fond of archetypal speculations to reflect a little on the definition of "solar plexus" currently found in modern textbooks of medicine, designating that particular sympathetic plexus situated at the level of the last thoracic and the first lumbar vertebrae. Doesn't this name "solar," reserved for an anatomic entity, suggest perhaps an astral conception in those first Western scientists who discovered the nervous structure of the plexus under their anatomic knives?

What power keeps the "material man" and the "astral man" united in a single individuality, only partially conscious of his humanity? Yoga replies: "the *prāṇa*." What is the *prāṇa*?

One can guess the meaning of this concept, so important in the whole of Hindu philosophy, by defining the *prāṇa* as "cosmic energy" divided into three currents of vital power: a physical current we can easily identify in all the forms of energy we know (electricity, light, sounds, ultrasounds, heat, terrestrial magnetism, solar energy), which obeys the laws of energy transformation; a biological current we can identify in the bioelectrochemical impulse that condenses into adrenalin and acetylcholin, once it has come through the nervous fibers; a third pranic current would go through man's entire cerebrospinal axis to nestle in the lower *Chakras*, that is, in the sacral and coccygeal plexuses, constituting a formidable supply of energy we call sexual energy, to which is bound the transmission of the human species, from individual to individual, from generation to generation.

So far, except for the names, there is no substantial difference between Western science and Hindu thought, such as the Yoga tradition passed on to us. On the other hand, what seems quite characteristic of Vedic thinking with respect to Western thought is the unitarian concept pervading the whole cosmic conception of which *prāṇa* is the concrete expression. Man is not placed outside the cosmos as a separate entity, watching the universe through his telescope or through his microscope to derive a few physical, biological, or chemical "laws" from it. Man, according to Yoga, is a microcosm, permeated, crossed, nourished, moved by the *prāṇa* exactly in the same way as the stars, the atoms, and the quanta of light are moved

The laws of energy transformation are valid not only for the different forms of physical energy, but also in the "integral man" the energy transformations are placed under the control of man's will.

If the cosmos could be compared to an ocean—says a Hindu parable—man can be compared to a wave. As long as the wave "thinks of itself" as a wave, distinct from the elements it formed from, it is but a small puddle of water stagnating on the sand, but when it manages to think of itself as a part of the ocean, then all the power of the ocean lies within it (Paramahansa Yogananda).

Yoga states that man has in himself a tremendous storehouse of pranic energy that he does not know how to use. By proper and steady training, it is possible to awaken the pranic energy within ourselves, to magnetize and to gain control of the *Chakras*. This goal achieved, it is further possible to bring peace and silence over the noise of our physiological networks, returning our three basic systems to an ordered and harmonious functioning under the rule of conscious volitions.

How this is possible through a steady practice of Yoga we shall discuss in the course of this book. But first let us consider for a moment the common man as he appears to us in his daily activity. He is a being in perpetual activity, constantly pressed by partly natural, partly artificial, impulses of every quality and quantity—sounds, lights, vibrations, emotions—to each of which he reacts by means of voluntary, habitual, or automatic movements. Even when his will would like to concentrate on a single object, keeping his body still, in reality his brain pays only partial attention to the object in question, since its sensory and motory areas are constantly disturbed by stimuli coming both from the external world and from his very "internal world."

Watch a young student at work, and take note of how many movements he makes with his hands, his lips, his eyes, his legs, and other parts of his body, yet appearing quite concentrated on his homework. Watch a man who states "he is relaxed,' and note his position, almost always spread over in the armchair or in the bed he is lying in. His disorderly attitude, even in its seeming stillness, involves multiple muscular tensions whose total adds up to an enormous unconscious and inefficient muscular labor. Even in his sleep, man often tosses, strains, and perspires, according to the rhythm of his uncontrolled dreams.

All this, translated in terms of human economy, means waste of biological energy. Through the nervous pathways, a continuous current of vital energy flows from the inside toward the outside, fading unused into the environment, supplying a very small efficient muscular labor compared to the consumption. The average man, because of his biological split, is an absolutely antieconomic machine requiring a great quantity of fuel to supply a very limited work. This happens in the normal man, but if emotive factors interfere, the consumption of energy climbs sky-high and can go bankrupt, burning and wasting the vital resources of the "vegetative" and of the "hormone" men who act as the watchdogs of life preservation. How many liver upsets, stomach diseases, heart ailments, how many headaches have this as origin of deficit because of foolish waste of energy?

Long before cars and television were invented, Yoga recognized the folly of man's useless race around himself. It analyzed its motives and indicated its remedies first of all in peace, in silence, in physical and in mental rest. Its message appears particularly interesting today in our artificial surroundings, which literally kill man step by step.

Is it all that simple, you would ask? It is not necessary to resort to Yoga to appeal to the usefulness of silence and peace. Modern man knows this and has tried to test its advantages. Newspapers and magazines are full of advice on the best way to relax, to "spend one's holidays in a useful way"; many companies are on the way to restore our environment to its original, unpolluted greenery; architects examine more and more rational ways to build houses impermeable to external sounds (except that afterward they fill them up with other sounds such as radios, television sets, record players, and the like). All our proud modern civilization cooperates to protect the human beings from the consequences of their artificial world, a world made of machines and gone mad in the noise.

The fact is that Yoga does not consider external, artificial means to bring man back to peace and silence, but exclusively internal means, committed to will and exercise. The difference is substantial: the Yogi does not need to go on vacation to relax. He can remain seated in a room open to the traffic of a busy metropolis and can transform himself to the point that he hears no sounds, being relaxed and quickly self-possessed on a chair, as if he were in a green Swiss valley. Translated into medical language, this capacity of voluntary sensory-motor inhibition is achieved through a gradual and conscious inversion of biological current: no longer a flux from the interior to the exterior, but a flux from the exterior to the interior. The Yogi learns how to stand still for prolonged periods of time in a correct postural position of complete rest, his vertebral column being quite erect. He learns to isolate himself from the external world by closing his cerebral circuits of sensory perception and motor reaction. Sensory stimuli still go along his peripheral nerves, but find the transit blocked at a certain level of his spinal cord or cerebral cortex. (See the "Spinal Gate" theory in Chapter 8.)

To give an example, again taken from electricity, the Yogi can voluntarily put himself in the position of a telephone or radio operator who wants to rest, and so switches off all the contacts of his sets: impulses still reach the sets, but are no longer perceived and, therefore, do not disturb the operator. Lying thus in a state of perfect and conscious peace, the Yogi can, through respiration, connect himself with pranic energy. Now he is like a battery put into contact with a source of electrical energy in phase of continuous charge, whereas a common man is like a battery working continuously, unable to recharge itself.

After he has isolated himself from the external world, charged with pranic energy, the Yogi gradually learns to make use of this energy to bring himself back into the original whole, sending the energy stored in the *Chakras* to magnetize the vegetative and hormone nervous systems. In his internal concentration, the Yogi feels his heart beat in a quite special and joyful way, until a day he will be able to control its rhythm, speeding it up or slowing it down. He feels the movement of his stomach and other visceral organs, and can put the digestive processes under voluntary control. He feels the blood flowing in his arteries and can increase or decrease his blood pressure. He feels the effect of the hormones and can control them, transforming them into psychological energy.

Thus, little by little, the somatic man and the vegetative man make friends again. The former learns to respect the latter, and stops pressing him with his excesses. The latter ceases to torment his somatic brother with his primeval instincts and learned habits. The third hormone man, since he is no longer compelled to work at a loss, can use his own hormone energy to the other two's advantage, by placing it at the disposal of his brothers' welfare. Very slowly, the three men learn to love one another and to identify themselves one into the other, till one radiant day they are ONE.

A healthy life in every physical and psychological aspect, a related training, a morality full of gladness and love, at all levels: this is how to attain the peace and the joy experienced by the Yogi when he perceives the conscious unity of himself. At this stage of his evolution, he is an "Integral Man," endowed with a great energy potentiality. He could spend this energy to acquire short-lived metapsychic powers, and so he would become a theatrical wonder and decay rapidly. Or he could guide his power to climb the peaks of *Rāja* Yoga, and become a mystic, a saint, always a master for mankind.

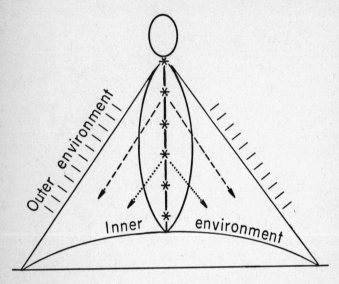

The three systems

DIAGRAM A On the physical level, human functioning can be compared to a computer, with three different kinds of "inputs" and "outputs." One set connects man with the outer environment (the somatic man); a second set of "input-output" connects man with his inner environment (the cells and the tissues of his body—the Vegetative Man); a third set provides the hormonal functioning. The vegetative and the hormonal systems sustain the vital and sexual functions, intereacting upon conscious and unconscious information received by all networks, through intricate and numerous feed-back mechanisms. As shown in this diagram, the three systems are connected through one common channel: the cerebrospinal axis.

Chapter Two

The Mind-Power:
Consciousness
and
Superconsciousness

The concepts "conscious" and "unconscious" have been expressed in the first chapter without being clearly defined in medical terms. Let us quickly discuss in this chapter the meaning of "consciousness" and "unconscious," as these concepts are currently seen in contemporary psychology.

Each human being thinks of himself using the pronoun "I" or the adjective "my." When we say "I" and "my" speaking of ourselves, we express a consciousness that we are living entities, somewhat different from other living beings. This consciousness is the result of the operation of the mind. What is the mind, then? Psychologists have many theories on the nature of the mind, but by no means have they reached an agreement.

We could think of the mind as an "organ of energy,"* a fantastic electronic system located within the brain. All the bio-electrical energy that we have seen continuously running down our nerves to the various muscles and organs is generated by the mind-power. The reversing of the out-going

*W. J. Bryan, "Religious Aspects of Hypnosis," Springfield, Ill.: Charles C Thomas, 1962. (3)

electrical stream into an inward movement through the Yogic training basically restores to the mind-power its otherwise dispersed energy, achieving as ultimate result an "illumination" of the mind itself. The "illuminated" mind in turn sustains those superior states of consciousness that I will soon discuss in the course of this chapter. At the time of death, the mind-power leaves the body as mental energy. According to the state of consciousness at the moment of leaving the "body-cage," the mind-power recognizes itself as "Ideal Man," a soul returning to the source whence it came.†

The human mind, although it is neither tangible nor can it be dissected like an anatomical organ *(we can dissect the brain, but not the Mind)*, is not less real than any physical organ, and its contents can be clearly tested and verified. If you doubt this, you can prove it yourself very elementarily: lock yourself in the silence of your room, recall an occurrence of your day's activities, then try to eliminate it completely from your thoughts. Unless you are already a superior being, in all probability the more you will try to shut that particular incident out of your mind, the more it will assail you with its emotional contents, pleasant or unpleasant as they may be.*

† The Greek word *psyche* means both "mind" and "soul." From the term *psyche*, the definition of "psychology" stems: Psychology—*psyche* + *logos* (discussion about the mind).

* In this connection, there is a fine Hindu parable: A man eager to attain occult metapsychical powers went to a famous Yogi and begged him to teach him the magic art of levitation. The Yogi smiled and replied that nothing was easier: "All you have to do," he advised him, "is remain locked in a dark room one hour each day, and think about nothing." "That's all," thought the ambitious man, "it's really simple." He was leaving when the Yogi called him back and warned him "especially not to think about monkeys." "And why on earth should I think about monkeys?" thought the man, and went home anxious to begin his training. But as soon as he sat in silence, trying to think about nothing, at once he remembered the warning received and told himself that particularly he should not think about monkeys. Alas, the more he tried to chase the monkeys out of his thoughts, the more these wearisome animals danced and rumbled in his mind. Three days later the man, humbled, went back to the Yogi and, upon the latter's inquiry, replied that not only had he learned nothing, but that the monkeys had danced in his rebel mind so long that he felt like he had almost become a monkey himself. (From: Paramahansa Yogananda's *Hindu Tales*, Los Angeles: Self-Realization Fellowship.)

We have thus evidenced a part of the mind, the so-called conscious mind where the conceptual patrimony gathered through the sensory experiences and their images and memories is preserved. From this source of memories, feelings, and thoughts our behaviors are ultimately derived. The interactions between the mind and the body in the life of relation form a functional unit which is called "personality" or ("ego").

The conscious mind, however, is only a small part of the overall, potential mind-power, a "little island emerging from the great sea of the unconscious," to quote a famous definition of the well-known Swiss psychologist Carl Jung, the founder of analytical psychology.

We have already seen that we are not conscious of our inner environment and do not have cognition of our visceral and hormonal functions. Then what is the "unconscious"? The unconscious can be defined as that vast area of the mind where concepts and experiences are preserved which have not yet been able to reach consciousness or which have been repressed by it. Jung distinguishes two forms of unconscious: a "personal unconscious" and a "collective unconscious." The former preserves all kinds of things forgotten, repressed, perceived, thought, or felt in a subliminal way, the latter hides contents that are no longer specific to our personality, and derive not from personal acquisitions, but from hereditary modalities of psychological transactions. The "collective unconscious," according to Jung's thinking, is a hereditary patrimony common to all men and perhaps to animals, and forms the foundations of each individual psyche: "Collective unconscious is more ancient than consciousness. It is the original datum from which consciousness comes always new; the new-born baby already possesses the unconscious psychic patrimony, and becomes more conscious the older he grows."

Having thus briefly outlined the definitions of consciousness and unconscious, let us take a closer look at the way we function at the psychological level.

First of all, contemporary psychology distinguishes three stages of mental development during our growth as human beings. The first stage, during early childhood, could be called a stage of "animal awareness": the child is conscious of his needs and wants, but he is not conscious of himself as a separate entity; he wants his needs fulfilled, but he is not prepared to give anything in exchange. The second stage could be defined as "lovable awareness," and is more or less developed during late childhood and early adolescence: the child learns to know himself as a separate being, with a body which has a head, a trunk, four limbs, different from all other bodies; he also learns to be "lovable," that is, to give something in return for the fulfillment of his needs and desires. The child may smile, may call "Dad" and "Mom," may be prepared to pay some little service to his parents, but basically he is totally ego-oriented, that is, everything from the outside world is expected to serve him, to play a function in his well-being. (How many adults really ever go far beyond this stage?) Finally, the third stage is currently called a stage of "self-esteem" or "full maturity," in which man learns to integrate the image of himself, made up of sensory perceptions, with the exercise of reason, in a well-balanced expression of emotions, based upon moral codes rather than upon selfish wants and desires.

Psychology recognizes that the above stages of mental growth are not fixed steps never to be retraced again, but rather plastic states of mental functioning that can be played over and over again during the entire life span. In other words, even when we have reached adulthood and psychological maturity, we are always exposed to a "regression" toward an earlier stage of development under the strain and the stress of daily living. A few examples might make the above points clear. If we do not steal, do not drive over speed limits, do not "cheat" while playing cards, and so on, in obedience to moral or legal laws and to ethical codes, then we perform as mature humans. But if we perform these same actions only in fear of being caught and punished, then we behave immaturely, in a way close to an earlier stage of mental development. If we work according to the duties that we have freely accepted with the job, honestly attempting to perform at the best of our capabilities, then we behave in a mature way. But if we do our work only to please our boss, or out of fear of being fired, then our behavior is certainly less integrated and more childish.

It is obvious that each one of us is likely to behave in mature or immature ways, according to the interplay of numerous and interchanging factors in the familiar and social environment.

For instance, few of us might cheat at cards, but how many of us would observe the highway speed limits if we were sure that no police patrol was scouting around? Failures to grow substantially mature, failure in our moral functioning, are known to be at the very source of most of those mental disorders expressing themselves in neurotic behaviors, such as hysteria and compulsive obsessions.

Our mental functioning is based upon a number of different factors in close relationship with each other: (1) the sensory data reaching the brain centers via the sensory nerves, from the sense organs all the way up; (2) the perception of the sensation; (3) the evaluation of the perception; (4) the reaction to the sensory perception, after it has been evaluated. Again, some examples may help us to grasp these concepts. When we go to attend a concert, we receive a number of sound waves (the sensory data) that we perceive as harmonic music. Then we evaluate this music not only as it is, but also in relation to its meaning for us, to past memories, to the social environment we live in, and so on. This evaluation of the music generates our response to it, which may be keen attention, somnolence, restlessness or immobility, that is, different reactions to the same sensation. If we hurt ourselves while playing football, we will perceive the hurt as an unpleasant sensation, but we will also quickly evaluate it in connection with the game we are in. Our reaction to the hurt, therefore, will be dependent not only upon the painful perception, but also upon its evaluation. This latter will probably be a determining factor in our further performance during the game.

The sensory perception is usually evaluated along three main lines: (1) a line of emotional feelings, in terms such as "like-dislike," "pleasant-unpleasant," "good-not good," etc.; (2) a line of rational processes, such as "true-false," "right-wrong," "being-not being," and similar; (3) a line of intuitive activity, where the sensory data are perceived and evaluated in terms of the potentialities inherent to the physical phenomena. In other words, the so-called "intuitive perception" does not look at the phenomena in their sensory details (shape, color, smell, material of construction, etc.), but rather is capable of seeing at once the intimate nature of any given physical phenomenon, its connections with others, and the possibilities inherent to the whole. For instance, where the majority of people will see only a flower, with its beautiful color and scent, the man of intuition will discover the connections of the flower with the plant, with the soil, with the vegetal and animal life all around; he will be able to see similar flowers in similar plants. and to perceive intuitively the relationship between their inner natures. Intuitive perception becomes "pure intuition" when it no longer works on sensory data but on abstract concepts, such as mathematical symbols, in order to grasp the essence of truth over the limitations of our sense organs. (*See* Diagram 2) Creative works of art and science are mostly based on pure intuition, which may be later confirmed through laboratory eperimentation.

Man's psychological performances usually reflect all the three modalities through which we have come to know ourselves and the world around us. One of them may become predominant in the course of life, however, determining the ways by which each one of us shall be known. The predominant perceptive modality tends to develop and differentiate more and more as far as determining a "perceptual type" of individual: "emotional" (or sentimental), "intellectual" (or rational), "intuitive" (or empirical). Seldom, however, does one find perceptual types in one pure modality (in all Western philosophy, Kant is probably the only known example of a "pure intellectual").

From the combination of the three modalities of sensory perception I have just described, various personalities can be identified: (1) an "intellectual-intuitive type," whose form of thinking would have an intuitive character based mostly on sensory data: mathematicians, scientists; (2) an "intellectual-emotional type," whose thoughts would be turned basically toward the practical aspects of the world we live in: managers and businessmen; (3) a "sentimental-intuitive type," in whom the sentiment would prevail over the rational to support and develop the data from intuitive perception: musicians, poets, artists; (4) an "emotional-rational type," whose predominant feelings would be highly integrated with rational processes: physicians, magistrates, priests devoted to the practical exercise of their ministry.

Finally, our behaviors, that is, the expression of our meı tal functioning respond to three different factors: (1) cognition, that is, understanding of ourselves and of our position in the world; (2) volition, that is, the exercise of will power; (3) habits, that is, these binding forces that compel us to interact with our environment according to pre-learned patterns of behavior, repeated over and over again.

Our behaviors might distinguish us in two different classes of individuals: (1) The "extrovert," who acts according to external standards, collectively valid, following parameters dictated by his time and by the custom of the community he lives in. Consequently, he can easily adjust himself to the outer environment without too much strain. However, he is quite exposed to social manipulations and prone to be the victim of social assaults on his personality. (2) The "introvert," whose behavior reflects subjective criteria, that may or may not agree with the community's standards. The introvert can adjust himself with difficulty to a reality that does not meet his "ego's" approval. When the moment to respond to a particular circumstance comes, he usually withdraws, and only later, having absorbed the circumstance, does he react, not always in a predictable way.

In summary, our psychological make-up, our personality, is the result of a complex process of maturation. Familiar, social, racial, and educational factors play major roles, and ultimately determine our perceptual and behavioral modalities, which will characterize our mental functioning, once the stage of "self-esteem" has been reached. Man seldom knows how well adjusted his personality is, that is, he does not know how much he can "take" before his "self-esteem" will break down, "regressing" toward neurotic states. He is only confusedly aware of his predominant mental faculties, and his behavior is quite often dictated merely by habits, with little understanding and exercise of will power. Habits are tremendous forces that can be extremely beneficial in our total psycho-physical functioning—as a matter of fact, no one could survive without the help of habits—but they can also be painfully dangerous if maladapted or misdirected. A well-integrated personality should be able to watch continuously over the operation of habits, selecting them according to realistic goals and moral values, using them without being enslaved to them. How far we are from this ideal every one is free to guess, just thinking of *that* particular habit of his which he would like so much to get rid of, and which keeps coming back, bothering him with the force of its compulsion.

In the human consciousness, therefore, there are "points of darkness" and "points of light"—as Jung has called them. These latter reflect the degree to which man knows himself and is able to control his thoughts and actions. The "dark areas" hide those mental modalities of which man is unaware, and therefore cannot understand and control. If the environment and the type of job luckily fit with those mental functions that are "in the light," the resulting performances are likely to be harmonious and well-adjusted. On the contrary, a "wrong environment," that is, an environment or a job one does not know how to handle, will give rise to more or less conscious tensions, fractures between ourselves and the external reality, which constitute the basis for so many "wrong lives," and contribute toward the onset of numerous mental and physical disabilities.

What I have tried to say outlines the extreme importance for each human being to expand his consciousness in order to know himself better, and to understand the world around him in order to fit into it with the best chances of a joyous and productive life. In the words of Carl Jung: "In one's youth, the most important psychic task consists in developing that modality which, according to the individual congenital structure, can best be of use to him in getting a footing and responding to the exigencies of the external world. Only later—when youth is over and the adult age has reached maturity—can the differentiation of all the remaining mental faculties be started. Since every goal in life tends to totality, in one's psychological life it is also necessary to approach this ideal. If this need does not reveal itself at an early stage, the 'last call' sounds in the afternoon of our earthly life. One must obey it at this time or meet the evening of life tormented and defeated." How many of us, witnessing the anguish of troubled and tormented old people, the ravages of senile depression, have not evidenced this terrible truth contained in Jung's admonition, a truth that rests at the basis of the whole Hindu philosophy with its concept of "Karma" as cosmic moral law?

At the beginning of this chapter, I mentioned the "unconscious" in its two forms, "personal" and "collective." We can now better understand these notions on the basis of what I have briefly discussed about our mental functioning at the level of consciousness. We can imagine the personal unconscious as a voluminous filing system where we continuously put memories of past experiences, emotions, affects, perceptions, and thoughts we have repressed and removed from awareness, or that have never reached a conscious level. In a well-rounded personality, the unconscious is a vital reservoir of experiences to be used at appropriate times. For instance, in the face of a threat, we have available a store of unconscious memories of methods that have been useful in the past to cope with similar situations. Then we are likely to "search our files" until we find a memory trace of a prior situation where a threat was handled successfully.

However, the unconscious is not always a well-ordered filing system. Sometimes, it may be a dark and deep well where we pour the frustrations and the conflicts rising from a poorly integrated personality with a great deal of confusion and dark points in its mental functioning. In other words, the personal unconscious at least partially reflects the state of consciousness, and cannot be better than our personality is. In the physiological field, the somatic system usually imposes upon the vegetative system the consequences of many of its distorted actions. So too in the psychological field, a consciousness only dimly lighted discharges into the unconscious the consequences of its maladjusted and confused mental functions. The latter takes vengeance, producing discord and chaos instead of help, when requested to provide blueprints of past experiences. The intellectual who despises sentiment, the empiricist who stubbornly sticks to his intuitions, blindly refusing to accept the rational data, the introvert in an environment he loathes, the dogmatic without discriminative wisdom, all these personalities continuously provides blueprints for future unhappiness to themselves and their families through the misunderstanding of the personal unconscious.

If man does not believe in hell as a place, he would have good reasons to change his mind upon reflecting on the contents of a neurotic person's unconscious. He will then at least acknowledge the existence of hell as a psychological state of mind. As on the physical level, diseases and death are the result of the clash between the somatic man and his vegetative brother, so madness and suicide might await the man who has not been able to bring about peace in the clashes of his conflicts rising from a dimly lighted consciousness.

Collective unconscious—in the teaching of Jung—represents a patrimony of psychological experiences no longer individual, but common to the whole human kind. It consists of different ideational patterns according to which mankind has always acted since his beginnings, independently of historical and ethnical differentiations, in specific human situations such as the struggle against the forces of nature, the relationships between the sexes, between parents and children, generic attitudes toward hate and love, birth and death, darkness and light. In the collective unconscious therefore, are buried men's experiences, dictated by the two primeval instincts common to man and animal: the instinct of self-preservation and the instinct of reproduction.

Jung calls "archetypes" the fundamental ideas according to which, in the long run, men have built their collective psychology. This is something similar, I would say, to Plato's "ideas," that is, the "prime image," the "patterns of the phenomena." In the language of the collective unconscious archetypes appear in figurative and symbolic form. The motives of these forms and symbols are the same in all civilizations. We discover them in all the mythologies, the fables and the mysteries of a primitive religious character: Prometheus stealing the fire, Hercules killing the Dragon, Ulysses and Rama crossing the seas (of ignorance) in order to "attain virtue and knowledge," the myths of Isis and Osiris, of Jupiter and Venus, of the serpent, of the fish, of the sphynx, of the Holy Mother, of the bewitched prince, of the wizard, of the witches, of certain "fatal" numbers (three, four, seven, nine, etc.). These are figures and patterns of the "collective unconscious."*

* Unless we went to concede that Boccaccio and Chaucer, Grimm and Andersen, and before them, Aesop and Phaedrus, copied their fables from the tales in the *Pancatantra* or in the *Suka-Saptati* of Hindu literature, the remarkable identity of contents in certain tales of the *Decameron*, or of the *Canterbury Tales*, with similar stories in the mentioned Hindu

The archetypes represent formidable psychic powers, protective and beneficial vital forces when their values and their meanings are understood. In contemporary man, especially in our Western technological society, the archetypes have been distorted and deprived of their content, stripped of their original form by the substitution of political, social, and economic concepts giving rise to new "idols" (to use a Cartesian term) of materialism, nationalism, racism, and other such "isms." So we see how it is that man has been deprived access to his inner power, power he desperately needs to meet the eternal threats of nuclear annihilation, economic manipulations, upheavals, and even natural disasters.

As in human physiology man's three parts are kept together dynamically by a vital energy, this same vital energy pervades and connects all the forms and activities of the psychic system. In psychology, such an energy is called "libido" (*ojas* in the equivalent, exact Yoga language): it marks the intensity of the Mind-power and is measurable only through its effects. When set into motion, libido appears as the force of one's instincts, emotions, affects, and will power; of one's working and producing capabilities. In a normal man, however, only a small part of his psychic energy is at his conscious disposal, for the most part operating in the unconscious as a latent force giving a dynamic expression to unconscious contents. Often this force acts antagonistically to the force of consciousness, with damaging results to the entire psychological equilibrium. Useless dispersion of mental energy, unconscious and undetected, is probably at the root of many so-called psychosomatic disorders, manifested through various muscular tensions, which further deteriorate and waste vital energy. The results are seen in people who seem to be chronically "tired and worn-out," poor effort-makers, and chronic complainers of pains and aches.

In order to understand these concepts better, let us once

works, cannot be otherwise explained but by admitting an "archetypal" patrimony common to all mankind. This "world of ideas" common to men of all times offers an explanation for certain patterns of religious worship which can be found everywhere: for example, the concept of the Holy Mother as the symbol of natural forces can be found among the Hindus under the name Kali, among the American Indians under the name Mother-Corn, in the Christian worship of the Holy Mary, and so on.

more resort to a comparison taken from electrodynamics. If we imagine consciousness and unconscious as the two poles of an electrical system, connected one to the other with a difference of electric potentials, a current of energy will travel along the system, flowing from the area of higher potential to the area of lower potential. Likewise, in the psychic system, a current of energy flows from the area where a higher libido potential is present, to the area where the potential is lower. If this current travels in the direction conscious-unconscious, a psychological progress results ending in the complete theoretical illumination, which suppresses the disharmonies in the unconscious and restores man to his psychological totality. On the other hand, if the current flows in the opposite direction, from unconscious to consciousness, a psychological regression results, with more and more restricted areas of consciousness slowly submerged by the waves of the unconscious. The final outcome of this process unfortunately is more frequent than its theoretical opposite—the complete illumination—and is called "insanity," or death of ordered mental functioning.

Summarizing what I have tried to say up to this point, we can observe how physiology and psychology are in agreement in showing that the pronoun "I" and the adjective "my," of which we are often so proud when we think of ourselves, actually apply to a poor and small part of our totality.

On physiological ground, in fact, we are conscious—and more or less in control—of a mere third part of our total body functions, whereas in the psychological sphere only a smaller part of our mental functions is in the light; moreover, our own consciousness is but a small island in the great sea of the unconscious. I submit that the call to humility, a fundamental principle to any moral and spiritual growth, should start from this basic consideration of our inadequacy, which can be acknowledged on both medical and philosophical grounds.

Contemporary psychology considers man realistically as he is, with his particular ways of thinking and of dealing with life, and offers assistance and counseling in order to correct some mental disharmonies and to reverse some patterns of behavior into others that are considered better or more suitable to meet different problems as they arise. Psychology, however, and other Western sciences as well, while fully aware of

the imperfect nature of man, have little to offer for improving
man's evolution toward higher states of thinking, understanding, and performance.

Modern health and social sciences approach man from the
outside, and seem successful in providing him with better
health, a better education, and maybe some improvements
over his biological or psychological heredity. But in depth,
man always remains what he is, a small part of his physio-
psychological totality. It seems that the destiny of man is
sealed forever, never to be changed into something higher.
Millions of human beings are born, live, grow, reproduce, and
die at the same evolutionary level they were born. They have
gone through life without gaining knowledge of what the
human essence is, of what life is for. Thousands of others even
seem to go downhill on the scale of evolution, and become but
shadows of men, like animals observing the law of the jungle.

Hindu psychology looks at man in a different way. According to Yoga, man is a never-finished product of evolution, with
an endless potentiality for inner growth. The evolutionary
process has developed man up to a certain point and then
seems to have abandoned him. Further progress is entirely up
to the individual's will and effort. Like an artist, he can work
upon himself to make a masterpiece of his life, from the disharmonies and the noise of an imperfect machine to the
splendor of a "child of God."

Nietzsche understood this truth and stated that man must
be able to outdo himself. But his "superman" was conceived
upon an intellectual model, and not upon an actual spiritual
realization, and was therefore nothing but a magnified and
even distorted image of the average man: insanity was the
price Nietzsche paid for his mistake. Other philosophers and
thinkers, before and after him, understood human nature
better, and were able to go deeper inside. But they were unable to evade the feeling of dismay that the vision of mankind
as it is and as it could be usually produces in investigators
devoid of true spirituality. Any enlightened Yogi of India
would have been able to give a correct answer to such a
dilemma.

At the basis of Hindu psychology stands the same unitarian
concept I mentioned in Chapter One. Everything in creation

is a manifestation of energy at different rates of vibration. We ourselves—in body and mind—are nothing else but a particular form of the same cosmic energy, the *prāṇa*.

In Hindu cosmology, the idea appears of one indifferentiated "primeval energy" (in Sanskrit called *prakriti*) and infinite differentiated forms of the same energy, called *Purusha*. in Sanskrit. The idea of the *Purusha* can be compared to Leibnitz's conception of the "monad," that is, an individualized unit of intelligent energy. The Primeval Energy expresses itself according to three modalities, which the Hindu philosopher called *gunas: tamas, rājas,* and *satvas.* Once more, let us take a comparison from the physical world we know, in order to understand the concept of the three *gunas.* We know that matter can assume three different forms: solid, liquid, and gaseous, each one being nothing else but a different aggregation of the same number and quality of molecules. In a roughly similar way, *tamas* can be thought of as a state of energy frozen into dense matter, *rājas* as a semifluid, transitional state; *satvas* as a state of ethereal light matter, close to be returned to the primeval condition of pure energy. It may be a matter of reflection here to mention that in our language, the term "sublimation" means both the transformation of solids into gases and a state of mental exaltation in which we feel "lighter" and "elevated." Maybe the idea of the *gunas,* from the Vedic age, has entered in our archetypal patrimony, and still expresses itself today, semantically relating concepts of matter at higher vibration (vapors and gases) with ideas of mental elevation.

According to the prevalence of one of the three *gunas* in the human psyche, some psychological types can be distinguished. The "Tamasic man" is basically the common man, plunged into material life, with little knowledge of himself as a spiritual being, taken over entirely by the pleasures of bodily existence and by the means to secure them. The Western philosopher Kant has well described this psychological type— whom he defined as being of 'sanguine temperament"—in one of his less known but very keen "Pre-Critical Essays" ("Remarks on the Sentiment of the Beautiful and the Sublime"). In his quest for pleasure, the "Tamasic man" may turn to violence, violation of the natural and moral laws, until he generates a psychological hell within and around himself. Probably, at the lower levels of *tamas* the group of criminals of every kind, both from a moral and from a social standpoint, is to be found.

On a higher step in the scale of psychological functioning stands the "Rajasic man," bound for the assertion and glorification of his human personality on the earthly level, eager to get all the powers given to men by the human society: honors and glories of this world. *Rājas* is the "superman" of Nietzsche. In his stubborn quest for human powers, the "Rajasic man" may forget moral considerations, trample on the laws of human solidarity and charity, and thus regress into *tamas*. In so doing, he often triggers a kind of hell which is no longer psychological, but terribly real, such as wars, revolutions, economic crises, and the like. At the upper level of *rājas* are men like Julius Caesar and Napoleon; at the lower level lie figures like Attila, Robespierre, Hitler. The "Rajasic man" can be compared to the intellectual—predominant type at grips with his "light" and "dark" mental functions: a potential genius or a demon.

At the top of the human evolutionary scale is the "Satvic man," "the man who realizes the presence of *prakriti* in his *purusha*," that is, the man who is aware of his spiritual nature. Satvic is the man who aims at moral values; he is nourished by human ideals, he is sensitive to noble sentiments, to the duties and rights inherent to human nature. Within the limits of *satvas* stands the great group of artists, philosophers, legislators, scientists, who have done credit to the history of mankind.

It is important to understand that in Hindu thought, the three *gunas* do not represent fixed states of being, but rather outline the movement of constantly interchanging cosmic forces, in man as well as in nature. They also symbolize the various psychological personalities, such as each one of us is likely to be without any special effort, out of hereditary, educational, and environmental factors. Hindu psychology teaches that other stages of psychological growth above *satvas*, are possible, but they no longer reflect a natural process. Ascension above the state of *satvas* is possible only through man's supreme will and individual effort. The normal man "dies" when he reaches the upper steps of his natural psychological maturation, to be "born a second time" to the re-union of himself and to the life of the spirit.

Yoga introduces a new concept in psychology, which is now slowly infiltrating Western thought: the idea of "superconsciousness." In modern usage, superconsciousness can be defined as a state of consciousness where Mind-power is at full expression, all mental faculties are well integrated, and dark areas have been removed; where order and harmony have been achieved in the files of the personal unconscious, and the collective archetypes have been restored to their full meaning and value. Superconsciousness becomes "cosmic consciousness" when the entire individual psychopsysiological entity has been blended into a transcendental, intuitive comprehension, and our ontological, spiritual identity has been realized. In this exalted state of "total illumination," God is no longer an abstraction, but a Living Presence. The Hindus call it *tattwam-asi:* Joy, Bliss, Knowledge.

Almost a century ago, a Canadian physician, R. M. Bucke,* wrote a book *Cosmic Consciousness,* of which twenty-five editions have been printed. The book is quoted in the modern textbook of psychiatry, and its concepts are gaining an ever-increasing interest in the field of advanced psychology dealing with mystical experiences. In his book, Dr. Bucke has elaborated upon an experience of cosmic consciousness he had one evening in 1872, while he was walking home in a calm and peaceful mood, after a few well-spent hours with friends. In the *Proceedings and Transactions of the Royal Society of Canada,* Dr. Bucke's experience is described as follows: "All at once, he found himself wrapped around, as it were, by a flame-colored cloud. . . . He knew the light was within himself. Directly after, there came upon him a sense of exaltation, followed by an intellectual illumination quite impossible to describe. Into his brain streamed a lightning flash of the Brahmic Splendor. Upon his heart fell one drop of the Brahmic Bliss,

---

* R. M. Bucke, *Cosmic Consciousness* (25th edition), New York: E. P. Dutton & Co. Inc., 1962 (4).

leaving thenceforward for ever, an 'aftertaste of Heaven' ".*

Drawing upon his experience, Dr. Bucke has proposed an interesting evolutionary theory, which is close to Hindu thought and to the thinking of Teilhard de Chardin, as exposed in his well-known book *The Phenomenon of Man*.† According to this theory, human beings are going through an ascending, but natural, expansion of consciousness throughout the ages. From an earlier state of "simple-consciousness," or animal consciousness, where man was conscious of living, but not conscious of himself as an individual entity, we have evolved to our present stage of "self-consciousness," where we are aware of ourselves as beings separate and different from others. We are not aware, however, of our inner nature of spiritual significance and dignity. Elaborating upon his points with keen and in-depth observations, Dr. Bucke shows that the next natural evolutionary stage of mankind will be "cosmic consciousness." In it, the "Brahmic Splendor and Bliss"— today regarded as an extraordinary gift restricted to a few and elected people—will be shared by all the human race, when full awareness of our Spiritual Essence will be achieved.

Years later, Teilhard de Chardin viewed the same process of evolution as an ascent of love, considering "love" as a powerful cosmic force, capable of bringing light and "noumenic" knowledge to the hearts and minds of men.

Hindu cosmology looks at evolution somewhat differently, though basically along the same line of thinking, at least so far as this cycle of creation is concerned. The Masters of India teach that the solar system would periodically go toward periods of evolutionary ascent lasting twelve million years, then it would drift toward stages of involution of equal length of time, and then the entire cycle would begin all over again. Each one of these semicycles of twelve million years is called *daiba yuga,* and coincides with the different "eras" of human civilization.

* You may compare the above description with another beautiful experience of cosmic consciousness reported by Paramahansa Yogananda in his book, *Autobiography of a Yogi.* (26).

† P. Teilhard de Chardin, *The Phenomenon of Man,* New York: Harper & Row, 1965. (24)

As the growth of the different civilizations is affected, so too the human psyche feels the effects of the *daiba yugas*' alternating cycles. During the periods of highest evolution, men's psyche would enjoy the best conscious growth, and therefore, the greatest consciousness granted to men as "Sons of God," whereas during the periods of lowest involution, human consciousness would be almost extinct, and only the instincts would remain. Through Yoga, man merely anticipates his psychic evolution far above the *daiba yuga* he is called to live in. Consequently, those Yogis who have already attained *samādhi* today stand at a stage of consciousness normal men will be able to enjoy only within thousands of years.*

In its essence, therefore, the Yoga discipline could be considered an ascending path, capable of bringing man from his actual psychological stage up to the "Luminous Mountain" of cosmic consciousness, through different states of superconsciousness.

In his book, Bucke has indicated the following signs as proof that cosmic consciousness has been attained or is close to being realized: subjective light, moral elevation, intellectual illumination, sense of immortality and loss of fear of death, loss of sense of sin, feeling of awakening, the transfiguration of the subject as seen by others. I want to discuss these states of superconsciousness from the perspective of Yogic teaching.

Subjective Light

Probably one of the first experiences in the Yogic training is a unique perception of light, usually in the form of a luminous point or ray, concentrated between the two eyebrows, at the root of the nose. In due time and after effort, this luminous point expands like a rotating searchlight, assuming different forms with beautiful and ever-changing colors, until the entire body and the surrounding nature are perceived as waves of light. Yoga teaches that light is perceived as a direct consequence of the awakening of the *Chakras*, when the outflow of vital energy is reversed and directed inward, toward the vertebral column and the spinal cord, up toward the higher brain centers to "illuminate" the mind.

* Sri Yukteswar, *The Holy Science*. (30)

Moral Elevation

Also early in the training, the serious disciple will experience a change in his thinking and behavior. To his surprise, he comes to understand the true meaning of "freedom in morality," that is, the capability to behave not out of ego compulsions, but in a loving relationship with the entire Creation, according to universal values and goals. Nature loses its dreadful mysteries, and becomes friendly. The advanced Yogi actually knows that the essence of Nature is "love," and that this "love" works intelligently for all. Moral elevation can only stem from order and harmony within one's bodily and mental functions (see Chapters Three and Six). To the Yogi who has been able to tune himself in with the orderly purposes of Creation, nonmoral behaviors are no longer possible, since he himself stands up as a standard of morality. The great sages and saints did not deliver moral lectures, but moral côdes were written after their life patterns.

Intellectual Illumination

Ascending along the mystical path, the disciple gradually develops many latent intuitive modalities in his mental functioning. The fog of confusion that usually clouds our understanding, our cognitions, and our judgments is lifted, giving way to a clear vision of living phenomena. As a side consequence, an in-depth understanding of the esoteric teaching in the Holy Scriptures of great religions is gained; the Bible, the Bhagavad Gita, the Koran, become one great, single Holy Book, presenting in different words, parables, and doctrines the same Eternal Truth.

In time, "pure" intuitional powers are developed, enabling the disciple to rise above sensory data, and to know reality as it is, in contemplative meditation. Along with the intuitive potentials, discriminative wisdom is born out of the training, in order to properly interpret and integrate the data from intuition. (*see* Diagram B)

Sense of Immortality

At higher stages of the Yogic path, the Yogi realizes intuitively

his true essence, an intelligent, individualized Unit of Divine
Energy. This deep knowledge gives a tremendous sense of certainty; all fears of death disappear, since death is only a delu-
sion of our senses: divine energy can be transformed, but
cannot "die."

Loss of the Sense of Sin

Contemporary psychology recognizes that the sense of sin—
or guilt—is born out of failures in our psychological maturation. Immature people tend to isolate themselves in egocentric, selfish positions and attitudes, building up racial, social,
and national "idols" and "taboos," in order to protect and
justify their isolation. Psychology recognizes that the so-called
"guilt complex" is the most common cause of individual and
collective neurotic and psychotic behavior. Western religion
and Hindu thought basically agree with psychology when
they define "sin" as the isolation of man among his fellow
men, and of man from God. In other words, we "sin" when we
shut ourselves out of the stream of life, and fail to keep a
loving relationship with Nature, its creatures and Creator.
The sense of sin is shed only when man is able to come completely out of mental attitudes of isolation and selfishness, into
greater dimensions of love and unselfish behaviors. Superconsciousness and cosmic consciousness cannot be attained unless
we first learn to serve our fellow men with undiscriminated
love. The reward for service is loss of the guilt complex and
attaining the Bliss of cosmic consciousness.

Feeling of Awakening

Almost at the beginning of the training, a thrilling feeling of
electrical current is felt in the body, as the disciple gains control over his inner functions and brings silent peace among
his bodily systems. In more advanced stages, the "electrical
current" becomes "concentrated"—and is actually perceived
—along the vertebral column and within the spinal cord.
Finally, the advanced Yogic learns how to "liberate" the vital
energy—which is Himself—so to speak "channeling" it up
into the "ethereal spaces." This experience is felt as a great,
joyous awakening, as a glorious resurrection to the life of
Spirit, a Spirit known to be in ourselves.

The Transfiguration

The ascension to the mount of cosmic consciousness is also shown in profound changes in the outward personal appearance of the faithful disciple. The inner light seems to shine outward, gifting him with a highly magnetic personality, always of guidance and inspiration to others. Actually, people so fortunate as to come into contact with highly developed human beings detected and reported this "magnetic aura" around them. The "halo" around the heads of saints in the paintings of so many artists is a vivid symbolization of the light that transfigures the physical appearance of men in cosmic consciousness, as witnessed by observers throughout the centuries. The Gospels themselves bring testimony to what Bucke has written, in the beautiful description of the Transfiguration of Jesus Christ before the eyes of Peter, John and James, on the top of Mount Tabor.

Postexperience Behavior

Superconsciousness is a relatively stable state in which the developed Yogi usually dwells. On the contrary, only a few enlightened Masters are able to reach a permanent state of cosmic consciousness, continuously living immersed in its Bliss, so to speak. To most of those who worked their way up to the end of the Yogic Path, cosmic consciousness has come as a flash of infinite beauty, lasting only a few minutes. However, the experience has such intensity as to leave a permanent mark upon the man who has experienced it. Superconsciousness and cosmic consciousness reflect deeply in the way the disciple behaves in every-day life and interrelates with others. Our life cannot be divided into compartments; we cannot be "Yogi" in the morning and in the evening when we perform the *āsanas,* and then behave for the rest of our time in egotistic ways.

The fulfillment of the Yogic ideals is not only found in the conquest of higher stakes of consciousness, but also in a life of work, service, and unselfish productivity. The true Yogi, like every mystic, must be judged not by what he says about his beautiful experiences, but by the degree he demonstrates them in his relationship to others. The "transfiguration" is not only a matter of "auras" but also in his behavior, a behavior no longer tainted by ego limitations but rather universally service-oriented. Historians have recorded in the biographies of saints and sages from the East and from the West inspiring examples of lives spent in joyous service to mankind, following the ideals of Karma Yoga and Mystic Christianity.

Before closing this chapter, I would like to briefly outline the Yogic Path in its subsequent stages, in order to promote a better understanding of what has already been said, and of what will be discussed later.

The *Rāja* Yoga, according to the *Yoga-Sutras* of Patanjali, includes eight ascensional steps: *yama, niyama, āsana, prāṇā-yāma, pratyāhāra, dharānā, dhyāna,* and *samādhi.*

Yama. This first step comprises a number of rules the candidate Yogi is supposed to observe: (1) *ahimsā,* that is, nonviolence to people or to animals;* (2) nonfalsehood, to other people or to himself; (3) nonlarceny; (4) nonexcesses of any kind (food, sex, work, or luxury); (5) nonacceptance of gifts involving material obligations.

Niyama. The second step prescribes a series of actions the candidate Yogi is requested to follow: (1) *brahmacharya,* that is, purity of the body (in the physical sense of cleanliness and elimination of internal impurities) and of the mind; (2) he must be content with what he possesses and cannot wish for more than what is necessary to his daily life; (3) temperance and self-control; (4) zeal; (5) observance of the religious rites, faithfulness, and affectionate dutifulness to his Spiritual Master (the *Guru*).

Yama and *niyama* are essentially moral laws, which can be

---

* As is perhaps well known, the Yoga rule of *ahimsā* (nonviolence) has been raised to political doctrine, and was used as a method of social struggle by Mahatma Gandhi who, in his famous *Autobiography,* left us a document of what an Integral Man can do on the national and international political field. From Ahimsa comes the famous Gandhian law of "civil disobedience" according to which each citizen, "pure in mind and body (*brahmacharya*)," is authorized to disobey in a nonviolent way a law he considers unjust, and to request others to follow him in his disobedience. A proud Empire, the British, had to yield, and a nation of 350 million inhabitants achieved its civil and political freedom through such a doctrine. It has been said that only ten men like Gandhi today would be sufficient to solve all the social and political problems troubling our era, and to bring a just peace among people of every race and color. (10)

found, more or less alike, in any philosophical teaching of
ethical content, and in any religious discipline.

The Yoga teaching on morality, however, differs from philosophical or sociological morality in two characteristics. In the
first place, Yoga is not content with telling the disciple: don't
be violent, don't indulge in your pleasures, and so on, but
for each human passion, Yoga's millenarian wisdom has found
a remedy or an antidote. Against greediness, luxury, anger,
jealousy, the Yoga disciple is protected not only by definite
advice, but by exact techniques for psychophysiological victory
over his state of passion.

Secondly, Yoga morality is essentially a "pragmatic instrument" through which the candidate learns to tune in the
world on an active, and no longer passive, psychological foundation. The Yogi does not become elated with "beholding the
starlit firmament above him or the categorical imperative
inside him," as Kant did, nor does he lead a moral life in
order to obey the laws of his country or of the religious community he lives in. Much more modestly, he works on himself
in order to transform himself from a man of passion into a
man of morality, because he knows this is the first price, as
well as the first reward, on his way to cosmic consciousness.
When he falls down, he rises again, and tries to learn the
technique better. When he finally reaches the stage of *brahmacharya,* he is not affected by the moral results he has attained,
since he knows how long his journey still is.

Āsana. The third stage consists of a series of physical exercises, quite typical of Yoga, whose various purposes will be
better analyzed in a subsequent chapter. The art of the *āsanas*
constitutes the core of the Haṭha Yoga teachings, as mentioned
in the Introduction.

To remain within the limits of psychology, to which this
chapter is devoted, it could be pointed out that *yama, niyama*
and *āsana* aim essentially at raising man's psychological maturity to clearer states of consciousness by gradually developing
latent mental functions.

With the fourth stage, the Yogi decisively enters the domain
of superconsciousness. In literal Sanskrit, *prāṇāyāma* means
domain of the *prāṇa.* In its Yoga meaning, *prāṇāyāma* means
a series of techniques, partly connected to respiration, through

which the Yogi learns to control his Prana and to guide it at
will, to magnetize the *Chakras* inside. In the comparison of the
electric battery, *prāṇāyāma* would connect the battery to the
source of electric energy: through *prāṇa*, the Yogi is connected
to the Cosmos.

In the fifth stage, *Pratyāhāra*, the Yogi learns how to concentrate his pranic energy, channeling it up along the vertebral
column. *Dhāranā* and *dhyāna* lead to higher mystical experiences through prolonged and deep exercises of concentration
(*dhāranā*) and meditation (*dhyāna*). In *samādhi*, finally, the
Yogi enters Cosmic Consciousness and realizes the Noumenic
Reality beyond all phenomena in creation. In advanced
samādhi, the enlightened Master of Yoga, in a simple act of
infinite love, will reach direct and immediate knowledge of
God.

In synthesis, this is the "Luminous Path" of Yoga, ascensional, not easy, but *absolutely possible to each single man*, no
matter where he stands on the scale of natural evolution. The
glory of *samādhi* is open to all who are willing to make the
effort and to submit themselves to the guidance of a Spiritual
Teacher. Cosmic Consciousness is a deeply rooted birthright of
our human nature; indeed it is Human Nature herself as the
most exalted expression of Divine Creation.

At this point, we may ask ourselves: where can the average
man, the poor fellow of our big cities, harassed by a hallucinating civilization, crushed by the noise of a polluted environment, find the supreme will power capable of driving him up
the Mystical Path of Yoga? It is one thing in the peace of a
Hermitage among the majesty of the Himalayas, but it is an
entirely different matter on the streets of Paris or New York.
I cannot answer this question except deep in my heart where
no words can be spoken. However, I think that every Christian
can find an answer which could be called *Divine Grace,* and
every Hindu can find an analogous answer in his concept of
karma. Both ideas express faith in help from the Almighty in
return for deep and sincere "prayers of the heart."

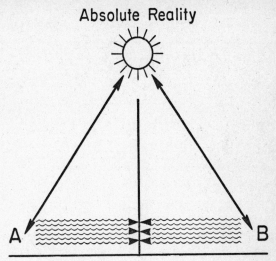

Absolute Reality

A   B

Human communication

DIAGRAM B   When A and B try to communicate with each other, it is as though a partial screening wall has been raised between the two. Each one of them will only see and understand a part of what the other is or says. Modern psychology knows well this "communication gap" and has indicated many of its factors, mostly based on failures in the sensory reception and transmission systems of both.

"Pure intuition" is achieved if A or B learns how to "tune in" with the Absolute Reality. Then they will be able to see and understand each other and all other created things as reflections of the one Supreme Reality. In other words, the Absolute shall act as a "Telstar" making communications among humans true and meaningful.

Pure intuition is no longer based on sensory perception, but on discriminative knowledge, born out of the same capability to "tune in" with Absolute Reality. Intellectual illumination in superconsciousness is the capability to see people and the world as "they are," and not as "they look like" in the illusions of the laws of relativity.

Pure intuition is gained not through any language, but through "silence," in what is called "contemplative meditation" in every Mystic Discipline (dhyāna). To those who know how to listen, "silence" does "speak."

Chapter Three

Energy and Foods:
A View
of Our
Nutrition

In the two preceding chapters, the concept of energy and the different forms energy assumes in coming from the Cosmos into the Earth, from the Earth into man, and becoming biological or psychological power inside man, have been mentioned.

So that we may be better able to face the problem of man's nutrition in following the thesis of this book, let us try to clarify our concepts of energy. What is energy? Opening a text-book of physics at the high school level, we find this definition: "energy—attitude of a system to perform a job; it can be *kinetic energy* when the job is being carried out, or *potential energy* if this attitude has not yet been turned into motion." Hence, according to the definition, energy is equivalent to movement. Everything moves and vibrates in the Cosmos, since every manifestation of the Universe is a product of energy; we are taught this law by modern undulatory physics and by Max Planck's quantum theory of energy, but the same law had already been told us by India's wise rishis thousands of years ago. Energy, this undulatory movement, pervading the entire Universe, can be discovered in matter as movement of atoms, electrons, protons, photons. Matter—states the Theory of Relativity—is but a particular state of energy "condensed in space" according to Einstein's formula: $E = mc^2$ (Energy = mass times the square of the speed of light). Living substance is a particular phenomenon of matter, endowed with characteristics of its own, but not escaping the great universal law: matter = energy = movement. In fact, everything vibrates in the living substance. Each cell composing the body of a living being on this earth is a microcosm where all the phenomena of the Universe are reproduced in miniature, and all are related to the formula $E = mc^2$.

An elementary Yoga experience awards the Yogi with a direct perception of the *vibrating movement* pervading the entire Universe and his same organism. As soon as he has learned the difficult art of complete relaxation and rhythmical breathing, at once he perceives a vibrating wave traveling along his entire organism like an electric current at a low voltage: he feels each single muscle, each single part of his body gently vibrating with a sensory perception among the most pleasant.

In nature, there are some great biological cycles in which certain chemical elements undergo successive transformations from simple into complex elements, and again into simple with relative energy transformation. Each of these cycles presents two stages—a vegetable stage and an animal stage. The vegetable (the green plant, rich in chlorophyll) plays a role of chemical synthesis forming an organic substance out of two or more inorganic chemical elements, storing up energy, whereas the animal plays a role of fission through which the complex substance taken from the vegetable world is decomposed into its elements, reduced of the energy it contains, and returned to nature. In other words, the green plant transforms the actual energy of the sun radiations into potential energy, and stores it as chemical energy in the complex organic materials it produces; whereas the animal transforms this potential energy again into actual energy, disguised as heat, motion, electricity.

Let us take as example the so-called biological cycle of carbon. Carbon is a natural chemical element, present everywhere in Nature in various inorganic and organic forms. Its molecule is made up of four atoms revolving around a nucleus charged with electricity. Using the water in the soil, the plant picks up

the carbon from the ground, and transforms it from a simple
element into complex organic products, appropriately called
carbohydrates (that is, carbon+water). The animal, feeding on
the plant, assimilates and separates the carbohydrates, utilizes
the energy thus released, and returns to nature the carbon, disguised as carbon dioxide (that is, carbon+oxygen—CO_2).
Other plants pick up the carbon under this different form, and
again join it to the water in the soil to form carbohydrates,
while the oxygen is again readmitted into the atmosphere, at
the animal respiration's disposal.

The operation through which the green plants are capable
of picking up the carbon dioxide is well known under the
name chlorophyll photosynthesis, since it is entrusted to the
granules of chlorophyll present in the green parts of the plants,
under the influence of sunlight, which supplies the needed
energy. Other biological cycles fundamental to the animal life
are those of nitrogen, sulphur, and oxygen, all three requiring
the presence of the green plants. Hence comes the archetypal
cult of "Green Nature." Here lies the scientific justification
for wholesome walks in the woods, for green parks instead of
polluted cities. Here, in its biological capacity, reappears the
ancient Yoga advice of a quiet life in hermitages among forests
and woods at the foot of the mountains.

Therefore, man and animal are energy transformers, that is,
they are motors. The definition of motor currently given for
the human body must not, however, create confusion. Man's
body functions like a motor, but man is not a motor. A Spirit
lies within man which does not obey the laws of physics,
although many correlations exist between the two entities.

Like every motor, the human body requires the presence of
two elements for its operation—a combustible element and a
burning element. The latter is Oxygen, the only burning substance present in the earth's atmosphere, which is inhaled in
the body through respiration. On the other hand, the fuel is
supplied by the manifold variety of foods reaching man from
the vegetable and the animal kingdoms through culinary art,
mastication, and swallowing of the chewed food. The swallowed foods reach the stomach and the intestines, to undergo
complex chemical transformations which, on the whole, in
medicine are given the name metabolism. The transformation

of the potential energy enclosed in the foods into actual energy (thermic, mechanical, electrical energy, and so on) constitutes the so-called energy metabolism, whereas the elaboration of the nourishing principles into cellular material, that is, into organic substances needed by the cells and tissues of the body, constitutes the so-called material metabolism.

Energy Metabolism

In every aliment are present various chemical substances—carbohydrates (otherwise called sugars), fats, and proteins (animal and vegetable). The specific amount and quality of each of these substances differs from food to food. Fruits and vegetables are rich in carbohydrates, but have almost no fats. Meats and eggs are rich in proteins and fats, but poor in carbohydrates. Milk has all three of the substances in a balanced proportion; cereals are rich in proteins and carbohydrates.

Yet carbohydrates, fats, and proteins are combustible substances that release various amounts of energy, as they burn. In human physiology, this energy can be computed on the basis of the amount of oxygen used up to feed the combustion. The ratio between carbon dioxide production and oxygen utilization is called the Respiratory Quotient (RQ). The respiratory quotient represents a precise datum of the potential energy value of the chemical substances present in the foods we eat—for carbohydrates it is 1, for fats it is 0.7, for proteins it is 0.8. This means that, burning, a gram of sugar is completely transformed into energy, but that a gram of fat or protein does not burn entirely, and partially ends in smoke, that is, it produces dross that has to be eliminated. The removal of protein and fat dross, that is, those substances barren of energy, which remain in the blood after the combustion of proteins and fats, occurs almost exclusively through the kidneys as urine.

Therefore, from this simple observation, it is obvious that a diet rich in proteins and fats (meat diet) imposes hard work on the kidneys during the span of a lifetime. Hence many diseases, so-called Metabolic diseases, are due to the progressive accumulation in the blood of substances that the kidneys were not able to eliminate, either because they were fatigued, or because they were sick themselves; a typical metabolic disease is the gout. The lesions hitting the arteries in atherosclerosis and in other diseases of the circulatory system are undoubtedly related to a diet abounding in meat and animal fats. Recent medical studies have definitively tied our diet with the onset of atherosclerosis. In one of these long-term investigations, a group of monkeys was fed with a "typical American diet" and another group with a "low-cholesterol diet." Within two years, in most American diet animals gross atherosclerotic lesions were discovered, whereas little disease developed in the monkeys fed with low-cholesterol diet. The so-called American diet offered eggs, meat, and dairy fats, while the low-cholesterol diet offered no eggs and a marked decrease in the quantities of animal and dairy fats.

By supplying the utmost potential energy, a gram of sugar makes all the foods rich in carbohydrates better apt to render fast and efficient energy service. Everybody certainly knows the benefit of a few lumps of sugar taken at a time of extreme fatigue and cold weather. The alcohol contained in so-called alcoholic beverages is but a distillate of fruit sugars, and therefore constitutes a good energy nutriment. This benefit, however, is often spoiled by the disturbing effects overindulgence of alcohol exercises on the nervous system, as anyone who has ever been "blind drunk" in his life well knows.

The energy liberated from the foods is utilized to feed two different processes: (1) to provide for the working of the vital organs (heart, lungs, liver, kidneys, and so on); this energy is called basal energy, providing for the so-called basal metabolism; (2) to provide for the muscular work, enabling the individual to move around in his surroundings. Referring to the symbolic figuration in Chapter One, we could say that basal energy is the energy required to keep the vegetative man alive, whereas all the rest is awarded to the somatic man. Thus it is clear that if this latter uses up too much energy in order to move, work or enjoy exceedingly, while the energetic capital placed by nutrition at the organism's disposal remains the same, his poor vegetative brother will be at his last gasp, unless the alimentary input is increased. Even if this is justified in particular cases (very heavy jobs, sporting contests, and the like), it is indubitable that a too abundant nourishment in a lifetime prematurely wears out the liver, the kidneys, and the arteries, especially if this nourishment consists primarily in meat and savory fats.

There is more. Today we know that the taking of foods alone causes an increase of metabolism, partly to supply the energy necessary to the digestive processes, partly because of a so-called "dynamic-specific action" of foods, particularly marked by the presence of proteins, on whose intimate causality light has not yet completely shed. Thus a vicious circle is caused, which is among the sliest vicious circles of a man's life. The excess of energy consumption in the system of relation makes necessary an alimentary increase. In turn, this food increase raises the energy demands unproportionedly, so that the amount of food tends to increase, and requires a disproportionate waste of energy for its own digestion and assimilation. Thus, metabolism climbs and clashes with the real consumption needs of the individual. The "drosses" accumulate, the arteries harden, and one bad morning, the heart goes on strike, resulting in an "infarct." How many compulsive workers, how many jovial, hearty eaters, perfect drinkers, seemingly endowed with health and an enviable appetite, have ended this way. Consider that during elaborate digestions nearly all of the caloric consumption of the human organism, about 3,000 calories, is spent in assimilative and digestive needs. You can readily see the absurdity of an engine that feeds on fuel for the only purpose of burning it, without getting any work in return from it and without any production of energy except in the form of heat. Yet this is the result, almost to the letter, of hyperalimentation.

Material Metabolism

Each of the substances we call carbohydrates, fats, and proteins possesses a particular structural formula of its own. We can imagine a "structural formula" as a construction made up of small cubes: by changing the arrangement of the small cubes, the construction changes, even if the material and the number of the small cubes is exactly the same. The "small cubes" of our example are the simple chemical elements combined one with the other to form the complex construction of the protein, fat, and sugar molecules. The chief small cubes forming the alimentary substances are four—carbon, hydrogen, nitrogen, and oxygen. Their constant presence inside living matter has determined the appellative "organic substances" for those substances containing them. Organic substance is found in Nature and makes up the human body, but the arrangement of the small cubes changes. In chemical terms, the structural formulas are different in the alimentary proteins, fats, and carbohydrates, and in the cells of the human tissues. To decompose the chemical structure of the aliments is the task of digestion, entrusted to the juices of the stomach and of the intestines. To reassemble new constructions, chiefly protein compounds, from the disassembled elements, is the task of assimilation, which occurs mostly inside the liver. These two stages, digestion and assimilation, together constitute an important part of material metabolism, called the "anabolic phase."

But the human body is not a static building, like a house or a bridge. It is a dynamic organic formation, in continuous movement of energy and plastic transformation in accordance with the universal laws of energy versus matter. The cells and tissues forming our body are continually renewed after they have been consumed, either because of working needs, or because of wear and tear. On the material level, chemically speaking, we "die" every instant, and every instant we rise again with new cells and tissues. This aspect of metabolism, which embraces the destruction or transformation of cellular components, is defined as the "catabolic phase."

The liver is a highly specialized chemical power plant, a vast and flawless laboratory in charge of the transformation of the organic substances into the anabolic or catabolic phases. This great organ receives from the blood the small cubes that were disassembled in the stomach and in the intestines, and reassembles them into new organic substances, into new materials quite similar to those which have been destroyed within the tissues and are being replaced. If the anabolic and catabolic phases counterbalance each other, the liver's work will be limited. If, on the contrary, catabolism prevails, the liver will have to work at a faster pace in order to replace the losses. In the opposite case, that is, when the anabolic prevalence occurs, the liver will still have to work in order to transform the unused material into fats, to build up a plastic and energetic reserve. Up to a certain point, this fat reserve is useful to the general economy of the body, but more than necessary may become harmful, as is the case in chronic obesity. Catabolism increases during bodily and mental activity, and decreases during periods of rest; anabolism prevails during rest to restore the material consumed during the exertion.

The whole process of nutrition, especially the work of the stomach and liver, is made easier when the alimentary substances have a structural composition already similar to that of the human tissues. On the other hand, the process is made all the more complex when the ingested foods are structurally different from the tissue components. For example, among all the nutriments, milk is the only one that contains sugars, proteins, and fats in fair proportions, with structural formulas close to those of the human tissues. Besides milk, the proteins contained in meat have structural formulas close to those of the proteins contained in human muscles.

Therefore, material metabolism provides for the maintenance of the body and the preservation of the individual by using the energy supplied by energy metabolism. Both work on the nutritive elements ingested with the foods. But nutrition not only satisfies the needs of the individual, its usefulness is also extended to the very preservation of the species, through the alimentary energy transformed into sexual energy.

Individual preservation and reproduction are strictly connected phenomena. An alimentary deficiency is followed sooner or later by a sexual deficit, or just as soon by the failure of the fecundative capability in man, or of the ability to become pregnant in the woman. The equation is reversible, in the sense that an alimentary excess often marks a sexual excess. In the animal, the preservation and the reproduction instincts are harmoniously guided, so that the animal takes in the food that best suits him for quantity as well as for quality, just as his sexual stimulus is adapted to the needs of the species to which the animal belongs. In man, irregular and discordant as he is, the instincts have ceased to function as regulating elements, and have yielded their place to more or less unhealthy habits, if not quite to compulsions and sense-slavery. Gluttony leads man to hypernutrition, which slowly kills him on the physical level through a progressive deterioration of the liver, stomach, kidneys, and arteries; just as sex lust, gluttony's twin sister, kills man's consciousness through the obscure forces of the unconscious. When religious precepts censure gluttony, and require some "alimentary penance" on holy days before any other consideration, they want to recall man to these fundamental biological truths.

Besides organic substances in his diet, proteins, fats, and sugars, man needs other substances able to satisfy other necessities, no longer plastic and energetic in character, but osmotic. These are water and inorganic salts. Seventy-five percent of the human body's weight is made up of water and salts in watery solution. This water and these salts are divided into two great partitions—an extracellular compartment embracing all the spaces between cells inside the human tissues as well as inside the arteries, the veins and the lymphatics, and an intracellular compartment properly constituting the protoplasm, the same substance of which the cells are made. Between the two spaces, the extracellular and the intracellular compartments, a continuous movement of water and salts is carried on, following the biophysical laws of osmotic pressure. The inorganic salts in solution are numerous, but the most important of them certainly is sodium chloride. In fact, even a modest deficiency of sodium chloride in a man's diet involves the rising of a tormenting thirst much greater than the simple thirst for pure water, as anyone can verify by observing the severe thirst that arises after a severe sweat. (Perspiration is highly salted water.)

Repeatedly we have compared the human body to an electric battery. We can now see that such a comparison is not merely imaginative but reflects a biological reality. For the two compartments, extracellular and intracellular, work like the cells of a battery. Schematically, everybody knows how a battery runs: There is a fluid, distilled water, in which some electrolytes are placed in a solution. When an electrical current runs through the distilled water, these electrolytes gather around one of the two poles of the battery which is thus "polarized" or "charged." When the current ceases to flow, the electrolytes turn again into a solution, gradually releasing the electrical energy stored during the polarization; at the end, the battery will be depolarized or "run down." A similar phenomenon occurs in the human body: When a bioelectrical current runs through it, the electrolytes in extracellular solution are transferred into the intracellular fluid and energize the protoplasm. When the bioelectrical current drops, the flux reverses, and against the electrolytes return into the extracellular spaces, discharging current. The life of the cells and tissues is a continuous ebb and flow of this kind. When the flux ceases, life ceases, the cells and tissues die, the entire organism dies.

To complete this outline of human nutrition, we shall recall still some more elements which, in spite of their small number, play a qualitative role fundamental to the vital equilibrium of the human organism. These are a few inorganic chemical substances, metals and metalloids, the "oligo-minerals," and vitamins. Both reach man prevailingly through fruit and fresh vegetables. We can picture the oligo-minerals and the vitamins as "quanta of biological energy," that is, material particles charged with energy that is passively transferred into the human body to reinforce energy metabolism. For example: Iron unites with copper to form hemoglobin, and a lack of iron causes some kinds of anemia; iodine forms part of the iodine hormone, and when it is scarce, goitre and hypothyroid cretinism appear; vitamin D is tied to the nutrition of the bones, and a shortage of vitamin D leads to rickets.

I would like to synthesize these notes on human nutrition by resorting to another comparison, this time borrowing from thermodynamics. We can imagine the human body as a boiler able to produce steam. The steam sets some turbines in motion, with the production of electrical energy resulting from the process. In turn, the electrical energy controls the work of the boiler, and causes some levers to start their motion (in the comparison: the limbs). The levers in motion generate heat. If we feed the boiler good fuel with a high energy standard, and if we control the draught exactly, we shall obtain a perfect combustion, with little smoke. All the produced energy sooner or later will be able, in thermodynamic effect, to be converted into electricity. But if we feed the boiler unsuitable fuel, or if we control the draught badly, we shall have a combustion with a lot of smoke and scanty production of energy. The smoke encrusts the pipes and reduces their caliber, the draught diminishes further, the smoke increases, and one unfortunate day, the boiler dies out. This is precisely the fate reserved for people who do not understand and who cannot control their nutritional needs.

In our example, we could compare the Yogi to a man who is able to use an atomic battery for fuel, and has furnished himself with a fuel supply of unlimited potentiality. If we want to thoroughly understand Yoga's position as regards human nutrition, we must look at the aim it proposes. The Yogi is a man involved in the most difficult of battles, a fight aimed at bringing back to Consciousness and Unity the divided parts of himself. For such a task, he needs vital energy, not the simple energy for his everyday life, but a formidable patrimony of energy, a great deal more than the amount an average individual can yield without careful training. In the *yama* and in the *niyama*, the first two stages of the Yoga training, are contained rules of practical life, perfectly valid even for nutrition: "continence" and "nonviolence" (*ahimsā*).

Let us examine these rules of the Yoga discipline, as they apply to nutrition, according to the concepts we have tried to clarify in this chapter.

First of all, one must cut down on the unnecessary or useless waste of energy. The Yogi will start by feeding his body only as much fuel as he feels is adequate for a perfect combustion and nothing more, properly adjusting his "draught," so as to produce the most energy with the least work and waste. In practice, this can be achieved by three means: quantitative reduction of the alimentary volume (never fill one's stomach beyond a third of its capacity, always rise from the dinner table with a residue of appetite—these are golden rules of hygiene with a universal value); qualitative food reduction, giving the preference to those nutriments presenting the lesser "dynamic-specific action"; catabolism reduction through a balanced life, led in orderly work, disciplined rest, peace of mind. By reducing the catabolism and the food intake, the anabolic necessities are automatically reduced, energy metabolism goes down to an almost basal level, the speed of combustion slows down and improves, so that the food intake, insufficient to the average individual who leads an immoderate life, becomes sufficient and efficient to the Yogi. The set of these precautionary practices falls within the generic law of "alimentary continence," whose enforcement, before being a religious precept, is a sound rule of sanitary living, in harmony with the physical laws of the Universe.

Secondly, the Yogi should "purify his body," that is, he should reduce his combustion slags by increasing the energy production without increasing the fuel input. This he can do through a careful selection of his food. It was mentioned that a gram of sugar burns entirely with no slags. This chemical characteristic is enough to prescribe many sugars as nutriments in a Yogi's diet. Now, sugars are contained in the pulp of fresh fruit, an abundant nutriment in a Yogi's diet. Secondly, it was observed that the anabolic work of the liver to produce cellular material is made all the easier when the nutriment is structurally similar to the human tissues. It is maintained, and would seem at first sight, that the meats, especially beef, highly comply with this qualification. In reality, things are a little different when one ventures somewhat deeper than appearances of such hasty statements, as Yoga does in its most ancient experience. There is no question that "fresh" beef and veal are structurally similar to the human flesh, but what can be said of the same meat after the first hours following the animal's death?

Biology teaches us that as soon as life ceases, the animal proteins "coagulate" within a few hours, that is, they "methylate"; their original structure goes to rack and ruin, and is replaced by other structural formations quite dissimilar from the protein make-up of the living animal. These new denatured proteinous substances are called "ptomaines," and constitute the toxins of putrefaction. Not only does man regularly eat meat preserved for at least a few days, he intentionally lets it become tender in the refrigerator, whereby its taste and tenderness is improved. Then what does he eat at table with his fine, juicy steaks? Very little of the original beef proteins. Instead, he swallows many more ptomaines, and entrusts to his poor liver the care of rebuilding from this waste material new and genuine proteins, useful to the human tissues.

Yoga rallies good biological arguments against a meat diet. The fact that originally man was not a carnivore would seem to be demonstrated by the different constitution of his teeth and intestines, compared with those of a genuinely carnivorous animal. In the latter the incisors are little developed, whereas the canine teeth are very long to enable the animal to sink into its prey and immobilize it, and the molar teeth are pointed so that the animal can separate and chew the various fibers of the meat a little bit better. Man's set of teeth is very different, with developed incisors, reduced canine teeth, flattened molar teeth. The intestines of a carnivorous animal, measured from mouth to anus, is about 3 to 5 times longer than its body, whereas in man, the length of the intestines is barely double and approaches rather the length of the intestines of a frugivorous animal.*

The Yoga Doctrine presents other arguments against the use of meat, which are not of a strictly medical nature; these shall be mentioned here to close the subject persuasively.

We know from physics that solar energy lies at the origin of all the vital phenomena occurring on our Earth. This same solar energy is stored in potential form inside the green plants and their fruits. When man feeds on fruit and vegetables, he assumes direct solar energy. In other words, he feeds on "live" food, just picked, which he can swallow raw or just cooked with little seasoning, rich in vitamins and oligo-mineral elements, additional sources of vital energy. But when man feeds on meat, he swallows "dead" food in every sense, food from which vital energy is, so to speak, picked second-hand, after it has already been incorporated within the body of the herbivore, man's favorite prey. Vegetables and fruit, perfect energetic foods, however, contain in scarce amount proteinous substances whose presence in the human diet is essential to man. In a healthy Yogic diet, cereals and ground nuts, eventually supplemented by low-fat milk products, are suggested as excellent protein-supplying food, with low cholesterol levels.

Finally, Yoga resorts to one last argument against the use of meat in any man's diet. The argument falls within the metaphysical realm. The Yogi does not consider himself a superior being, uprooted from the earthly world he lives in, nor does he regard himself as being endowed with powers of life and death over the whole of creation. Very humbly he casts the roots of his human nature into all that lives—minerals, vegetables, and

* Sri S. Yukteswar, *The Holy Science*. (30)

animals. In his eyes, everything is the Work of God, and therefore has a sacred character whose enjoyment is allowed in the
observance of natural laws, of all natural laws.

The Yogi knows that all that he eats and drinks is taken
from some other life, small or big that it may be. He is aware
of the fact that the fate of innumerable vegetable and animal
species "goes through his mouth." Like a well-bred table com-
panion, the Yogi helps himself to moderate portions at the
great Table his Creator has prepared for him, and always tries
to cause the least disorder, the least destruction possible. Fruit,
vegetables, and milk do not involve any destruction of living
creatures.

This is the alimentary meaning of Yoga's diet regulations—
purity of body and mind, healthy food, "live" food, "pure"
food; a mind that is absolutely free of any thought of violence
against Creation, at every level of animal and vegetable life.
This is also the basis for the Law of Nonviolence: one cannot
be *brahmacharya* (pure of mind and body) without observing
the *ahimsā;* the *ahimsā* can be nowhere but in the heart of a
brahmacharya. The road leading to both goals runs through
man's stomach. Not at random does the Buddhist Doctrine
place the seat of wisdom in the stomach (whence the voluminous stomachs on the statues of Buddha).

Chapter Four

Energy and
Muscular Activity:
The āsana

A great part of the energy generated by the processes of nutrition during a man's life is used as electromechanical energy. A big consumer of energy is the activity of the muscle fibers. An adult man of average constitution, who is working at a regular, not too hard job, in normal environment conditions, requires about 3,000 calories per day; at least two thirds of these calories are spent to make the muscles work.

When we speak of "muscles," at once we are led to think of those fleshy formations we can feel through our skin. Those are the so-called "somatic" or "striate muscles," and belong to the system of relation: they are called voluntary because they more or less obey the brain's commands. But there are other muscles, in a much greater number, which constitute the structure of the heart, of the stomach, of the intestines, of the bladder, of the arteries—these muscles are called "visceral" or "autonomous" since they seem to act in a quite independent manner, beyond the reach of one's conscious will. In fact, they are a part of the vegetative system—they are the muscles of the "vegetative man."

A physiological characteristic of the muscle is its ability to contract, which is also a property of the proteins forming the muscle itself, the myosins. However, the characteristics of muscular contraction vary a little from the voluntary to the autonomous muscles. Let us examine the details.

Each voluntary muscle is made up of a multitude of muscular fibers. Each one of these fibers constitutes an independent neuromuscular unit, and includes two parts: a contractile part, and a so-called "neuromotor plate" formed partly by muscle, partly by nervous substance. This plate marks the junction between the nerve fiber and the muscular fiber.

When the voluntary nervous impulse reaches the neuromotor plate, it alters the electric potential present therein, creating a difference in the bioelectric potential between the plate and the contractile part, so that the latter contracts. Responsible for the change of potential seems to be acetylcholin, that microsubstance, that "biological quantum of energy" we have seen condense at the extremity of the nervous fibers (*see* Chapter One).

Numerous drugs are able to alter the muscle response to the contractile stimulus by keeping the latter out of the influence of one's will. Among these drugs, we shall mention two particularly well-known groups—curare and local anesthetics. Curare blocks the contraction at the level of the neuromotor plate, so that the electric impulse on its way along the nerve cannot change into mechanical energy, despite the presence of the acetylcholin. On the other hand, local anesthetics block the impulses along the motor and sensory nerves, even before they can reach the muscles. As it is perhaps known, local anaesthetics can be applied all along the course of nerves, from the spinal cord to the muscles. The closer to the spinal cord the local anesthetic is applied the larger will be the groups of muscles that will be blocked.

Muscular contraction can assume two forms. If the muscle is free at one of its extremities, it can freely contract with maximum work and a minimum of tension. For example, by contracting the biceps, I bend my arm: this type of contraction is called "isotonic." On the other hand, if the muscle is secured at both of its extremities it cannot freely contract, yet it is strained to its maximum degree. This form of contraction with maximum tension and minimum work is called "isometric." Example, contract the biceps while holding a heavy weight in your hand. In the untrained man, the two forms of voluntary muscular contraction co-exist: first the muscle is strained isometrically, then it shrinks isotonically.

The autonomous muscle has a slightly different structure. Here, each muscle fiber is not a neuromuscular unit, but the whole muscle is like a "rosette" of muscle fibers, without the motor plate, gathered around the point where the nerve fiber ends. The bioelectric mechanism of contraction is analogous to that of the striate muscles, although in many autonomous muscles, especially in those of the arteries, the microsubstance condensed by the nervous impulse is not acetylcholin, but adrenalin (nor-epinephrine). Just as the voluntary muscles are controlled by the motor nerves of the somatic system, so the visceral muscles are controlled by the nervous fibers coming from the various plexuses of the vegetative nervous system.

At the beginning of the chapter, it was mentioned that muscular activity absorbs a considerable amount of the bioelectric energy produced by the cellular "batteries." In part, this energy is turned into "work," that is, into motion in the life of relation, and in part, it is transformed into heat, a reduced form of energy, no longer capable of transformation. We could picture how the "muscle machine" works in this way. The bioelectric impulse starts a chemical reaction, which will release the potential energy contained in the muscle proteins, by using the fuel supplied by the sugars stored in great quantities within the muscles. If the contraction has an isotonic character, a production of work will result. If, on the other hand, it has an isometric character, it will be transformed into heat. If one lifts up an arm, he will produce a work; but if one tries to lift an arm while holding a heavy weight, less work will be produced with the same amount of energy, and sweat is likely to follow. Sweat, in turn, is a biological reaction to increased heat production.

In the normal man, the striate and the autonomous muscles rarely are in a state of complete rest. Within them always persists a certain variable degree of tension, called "basal tension" or "muscular tone." In part, this represents the elastic properties of the muscle fibers, which are related to the structure of myosin itself, but in a greater part it is the consequence of nervous impulses constantly arriving from the nervous organs.

There are no qualitative differences between muscular contraction and muscular tone. The latter is nothing but a subliminal isometric contraction, present both in the visceral and
in the somatic muscles. The basal tension is independent of
the common man's will. It is indirectly generated by stimuli
that continually leave the muscle fibers themselves, in relation
to their length variations. These stimuli reach the spinal cord,
hence they return directly to the muscle, in the form of bioelectric impulses. Such a reflex, which leaves out the cortical
regions of the brain, in physiology is called a "short spinal
reflex."

To understand this discussion better, let us picture the
mechanism of a spring. A spring can be stretched or shrunk.
But if we let it rest, it will assume a position that is neither
completely shrunk nor totally stretched. The muscular tone
can be compared to the rest position of a spring. When this
basal tone is upset, the so-called "spasm" appears. In physiology, spasm is defined as abnormal, involuntary, fibrillations in
the muscle fibers, which are often perceived as extremely painful. The elastic force of the muscular basal tension requires a
modest waste of energy in itself. This waste of energy becomes
enormous, however, when it is related to the entire surface of
the human musculature, and to the span of a man's life, energy
that disperses in the form of unused heat.

The basal tension of muscles can be temporarily reduced
through a few devices: (1) by stretching and handling the
muscle, in order to benumb the muscle fibers, in approximately
the same way that a spring that is stretched too much loses its
elasticity; the benefits obtainable through muscular massages,
designed to stretch the muscles, can be traced back to this
mechanism; (2) by blocking the nervous stimulus at the level
of the neuromuscular junction; (3) by depressing the spinal
cord, so as to reduce the spinal reflexes. The majority of drugs
we gulp down whenever we feel some pains and aches in our
muscles operate by depressing the nervous activity within the
cerebrospinal system (*see* Chapter Ten).

The muscular tone does not disappear during sleep or rest.
At the most it subdues, both during sleep and rest. When a
man declares he is going to relax, in reality he eliminates the
voluntary muscle contractions. He does not at all eliminate the

basal tension of his voluntary muscles, nor least of all does he relax his autonomous muscles.

Because of its functional characteristics, therefore, the human "muscle machine" is a totally antieconomical mechanism that can transform but a part of the energy it is provided with into work. Furthermore, it uses up energy even when it does not run. In other words, our muscles are engines that "heat" both while they run and while they rest.

No industry could afford to let such a machine run long, since quite soon it would run into deficit. In physiology this deficit is called "muscle fatigue," and each one of us knows how rapidly the signs of fatigue appear during even modest efforts. Muscular fatigue results from the rapid exhaustion of the combustible material ignited in the muscle by the nervous impulse, and by the formation within the muscular tissue of some substances degenerated from myosin, which constitute true fatigue toxins. Once these are removed from the muscle and the combustible supply is reconstituted through the contribution of new sugar by the blood, the muscle is again ready to operate.

Therefore, the fatigue phenomenon can be corrected in two ways: by reducing the basal tension of the muscle at rest, or by improving the working production of the muscle through training, with a better regulation of the burning and an accelerated removal of the fatigue toxins. The first method means a saving of energy, and is applied in the Yoga technique of the *āsanas;* the second method requires an increase in the consumption and utilization of energy, and is applied in sport training. In physiological terms, muscular training means to learn to reduce the isometric, thermogenic, contractile stage, in favor of a faster isotonic stage; thus the muscle becomes more plastic, springier.

In summary, autonomous and voluntary muscles do show similar anatomic and physiological properties, with moderate differences between them. In fact, both muscle types originate from similar embryological formations, which, only later on in their fetal life, will differentiate one from the other, according to whether they will form organs for the life of relation or organs for the vegetative life.

This common embryological derivation remains in the adult in that form known in human anatomy as "metameric arrangement." Without going too deeply into the difficult concept of anatomical "metamerism," we could picture the subject in this way: The voluntary muscles, which form the outer covering of the body, have close nervous links with the autonomous muscles, which are part of the internal organs, through connecting nervous relays in the vegetative plexuses at the same vertebral level. Consequently, volleys of nervous impulses from the spinal cord can fire at the same time somatic and visceral muscle fibers within close anatomical boundaries. These firings of both somatic and visceral muscles under the same nervous impulses is often referred to in medicine as "somatovisceral reflexes"; such metameric reflexes usually go unnoticed in the average individual under normal circumstances. However, when the rate of firing increases in either the somatic or the visceral muscles, that is, when the basal tension increases in one set of muscles, both muscular systems go into spasm and an unpleasant sensation is perceived.

Perhaps the discussion would be simplified by a few examples. Many of those who have suffered from acute appendicitis will recall that the physician visiting them carefully palpated their abdomen, causing a sharp pain at the lower right. The physician was looking for the presence of a viscerosomatic reflex, characteristic of acute appendicitis, whose symptom is a pain at the lower right side of the abdomen. At that point, the voluntary abdominal muscles are in spasm through reflex to a similar spasm hitting the inflamed autonomous muscles of the appendix below. On the other hand, those who have suffered from hepatic colic will recall the very sharp, excruciating pain on the side and back, characteristic of a biliary crisis. Here, the spasm of the autonomous muscles in the gall bladder has caused a viscerosomatic reflex in the surrounding muscles.

A similar mechanism causes the characteristic pain in the left arm and shoulder during the painful crises of angina pectoris. Still other people may have gained singular benefits in their digestive functions after a careful massage of the voluntary abdominal muscles. Here, because of the massage, the reduction of the basal tension, by somatovisceral reflex, has caused a reduction of the tone of the autonomous muscles of the stomach and of the intestines.

Muscular contraction is also greatly influenced by a man's psychological conditions. A well-balanced mind allows for a state of general relaxation throughout the muscular system, just as an unbalanced psyche, an unconscious too heavily loaded with conflicts, constitutes sort of a radiomagnetic station continually broadcasting jamming impulses. These impulses are "picked up" by the autonomous and by the voluntary muscles, which increase their basal tension until the painful spasm results; these are the so-called psychosomatovisceral reflexes. Many back aches and a great many headaches originate from an exaggerated tension of the muscles in the back, in the nape of the neck, and in the skull because of psychological tensions of various kinds. This fact has largely infiltrated the common parlance, and is expressed by phrases such as "to be tense because of grief," "to be tense awaiting something good or bad," "to fear so much that you feel the pit of your stomach shut closed."

We could also describe figuratively the concept of human metamerism as follows: The somatic man and the vegetative man are bound together by a dense network of relays all along the nervous system, in such a way that when one of them tenses, the other quickly responds with an equivalent tension.

Incidentally, we can note here that the concept of human metamerism, with its consequences of a practical nature, has been studied thoroughly and excellently applied in therapy, by ancient Chinese medicine for the cure of painful diseases. The needle therapy—or acupuncture—tries to influence the inner functions of the body through the insertion of special needles into specific areas of the skin. These cutaneous areas are located along lines that roughly correspond to metameric anatomic boundaries as Western science knows them.

Bones and Articulations

Up to this point, we have treated the muscles as anatomic and physiological units, and in our description we have associated the autonomous with the striate muscles. If the autonomous muscles are really independent units, constituting essential parts of the internal organs of the human body (the heart is but a particular muscle), the same discourse is not true for voluntary muscles. In the operation of the system of relation, these muscles are closely connected to the bones and to the articulations with which they form a single organic whole. In fact, muscles, bones, and articulations are but the different parts of a single "locomotive machine."

From the point of view of their operation, we can compare the bones to levers with a fulcrum in correspondence of the articulation, the force of the levers being applied at the point where the muscle inserts itself in the bone with its tendon. Let us take the example of the forearm with its two bones, the radius and the ulna. When I bend my forearm I make a fulcrum on the articulation of the elbow; I have a resistance in correspondence of my hand, and the force is applied on the radius and on the ulna, where the tendons of the flexor muscles are inserted.

In the functional economy of the human body, the bones therefore serve a double function—a static function of support to the mass of the body, and a dynamic function meant to improve the output of the muscular work.

All of the bones in the human body are connected one to the other through the articulations. The majority of these work like ball joints. The ball is made up of the round and smooth surfaces of the cartilages covering the articular extremities of the bone; between the two articular cartilages flows a lubricating fluid called synovial fluid.

The articulation is an organ exposed to enormous wear because of the dual, constant work it is subjected to during the course of its life. For, besides working as a mechanical joint between two adjoining bones, some articulations are constantly pressed by body weight. Think of the amount of weight the articulations of the lower limbs must support and move during an obese individual's lifetime. Things grow even worse when the man's carelessness further damages the articulation by leading an unbalanced life, or eating the wrong kinds of foods. Usually wrong positions of the human body, insufficient physical exercise, alimentary toxins, especially those originating from the meats, contribute to "rust" the articulations before their time, and transform a man, still in his prime, into a premature old man.

The rusting of the articulations is called osteoarthritis, and anatomically is characterized by a progressive destruction of the articular cartilages. When these cartilages gradually disappear, the two extremities of the bones, no longer protected by the articular surfaces, join together, and the whole articulation disappears. If the osteoarthritis—as happens more frequently—destroys the articulation of knee or hip, one day the individual finds himself in a wheelchair or in the dreadful immobility of a bed.

A particular example of muscularosteoarticular organization can be observed in the vertebral column. Anatomically, the vertebral column is formed by 33 vertebrae—7 cervical, 12 thoracic, 5 lumbar, 5 sacral, and 4 coccygeal. Each vertebra is a bone of a particular shape, with a hole in the middle and four articular surfaces through which the vertebra is articulated to the vertebrae above and below it. Altogether, there are 132 articulations in the vertebral column, four to each vertebra, two on each side. The set of vertebral holes forms the so-called vertebral space through which the spinal cord goes. At every level on the column, on the vertebrae are inserted muscles called cervical, dorsal, and lumbar paravertebral muscles. To these is entrusted the task of keeping the vertebral column erect, or of curving it according to the needs of equilibrium and locomotion. Out of the vertebral spine, through the so-called foramina between vertebra and vertebra, nerve trunks, variously combined into cervical, brachial, and lumbosacral plexuses, as well as forming 12 pairs of thoracic nerves, subserving the muscles of respiration. Each nerve trunk contains motor, sensory, and autonomous nerve fibers.

Moreover, to the thoracic vertebra of the spine, 12 pairs of ribs are articulated, forming altogether the rib-cage in which the lungs are contained.

The human body can assume countless attitudes, but three of them are basic: upright, sitting, and lying down. For each of these positions, the vertebral column plays an essential role. In the upright and sitting positions, it insures man the best equilibrium and walking disposition when certain laws are observed. Physics teaches us that the essential condition for a body to maintain its equilibrium is that the axis of gravity cross its barycenter. In the human body with an upright vertebral spine, the barycenter is based on the lumbar vertebrae (slightly higher in the man than in the woman) and the axis of gravity crossing a point along it forms a triangle formed by the two feet, slightly apart when the individual is standing, or is based on the perineum if the person is sitting. If the individual can maintain this position of natural physical equilibrium both when he is standing and when he sits, the strain on his vertebral muscles is minimum, and all the weight of his body is harmoniously distributed along the 132 articulations of the vertebral column.

But when an individual bends his vertebral column, he moves his barycenter forward, and the axis of gravity no longer lies between the tips of his feet when they are spread apart, or through his perineum, but is situated farther forward. Consequently, the static equilibrium of the body is risked, and a mending job must get under way to maintain the balance. This adjustment is carried out by the paravertebral muscles, which get strained to a point where the well-known back ache appears. Some people maintain that "with the inevitable back ache, man pays for the privilege of being the only creature on Earth made to live in an upright position." The statement does not seem fair. On the contrary it could be said that with his back ache, man pays for his refusal to live in a proper upright position, as he was intended to by Mother Nature, choosing instead to live and walk like an ape, with a customary position totally projected forward. But the ape is a quadrumane whose axis of gravity from its barycenter falls in a polygon formed by the animal's hands and feet, where man is not.

From this point, it logically follows that bed rest should, at least in part, repair the fatigue of the dorsal muscles. But it is sufficient to observe the way man usually rests and sleeps, literally spread all over his bed, or all cuddled up like a fetus in his mother's womb, in order to understand that sleep and rest are fictitious, and that on awaking, the back ache will be just as before, if not worse. In order to get a really good rest from our sleep, we should keep a relaxed supine position, as shown in Figs. 9a and 11a in the Appendix.

A correct position of the vertebral column in the three positions—upright, sitting, and lying down—is not only a question of good equilibrium and of rest for the vertebral muscles, but a precious requisite for a harmonious operation of the nervous system, hinged on the backbone and on the spinal cord, and for a physiological respiration connected to the rhythmic and free expansion of the chest.

Keeping the vertebral spine erect while standing up or sitting down has also an important psychological side effect. Physical and mental equilibrium are closely connected; it is difficult for a man bodily unbalanced to maintain a fair mental balance. Depressed people usually walk with bent shoulders and curved backs. As they stoop forward, the paravertebral muscles are chronically strained and aching. The chronic back pain in turn is contributory toward a progressive deterioration of the mental depression, in a dangerous vicious circle of psychosomatic illness.

Take note of the statues of the Pharaohs and of the ancient Egyptian priests in the Cairo, London, and Turin Museums. Observe the sculptures of the Assyrians, of the Babylonians, and of the Greeks in the Louvre and in the British Museum. Look at the attitude of the Emperors and of the Hindu Divinities in the splendid marble marquetries of the Taj-Mahal at Agra. Notice their perfect erect position, their vertebral column straight as a poker, in just about any plastic image they are represented. The ancients knew, better than us, the importance of a correct vertebral position as the prime expression of human dignity.

The Āsana

Āsana is a Sanskrit term which can be freely translated as "way of attitude." The Yoga position of *āsana* is, in fact, nothing but a particular plastic attitude of the body and mind, through which certain muscular groups are put into action and vitalized. We could define such statuesque attitudes as dynamic positions of the human body, statically maintained for a certain period of time; the set of these "positions" constitutes a static physical exercise with a vibratory character.

With the *āsana* the preparatory and purifying stages of the *yama* and of the *niyama* are past, and a sculptural, plastic process is entered, to lead man back to the re-unification of himself. In its tested experience, *Haṭha* Yoga states that, through the sole, regular, constant, and correct practice of the *āsana*, man is granted to climb many steps on the scale of his psychophysical evolution, that is, to go past *tamas* to *satvas* and hence reach the threshold of superconsciousness. Let us subject the psychophysiological secret hidden in the *āsana* to medical analysis.

First, I shall point out a few characteristics common to all the *āsanas*, and then we shall examine some of the more important "positions" in detail.

1. Each *āsana* involves a contraction of some groups of somatic muscles and the relaxation of their antagonists. For instance, when I bend my leg on my hip, I contract the leg-flexors, but I offer relaxation to the leg-extensors. By consciously pitting various groups of muscles against their antagonists, each *āsana* first brings awareness of the many faulty bracing efforts we make all the time with our wrong vertebral spinal positions; then it helps to break down useless antagonistic muscle overcontractions; finally it enables the disciple to achieve high levels of physical performance with minimal energy expenditures. Through the *āsanas* it is possible to reduce the basal tension of the muscles to a point that can be compared to the muscle-blocking effects of curare upon the striate muscular fibers. Just as it happens after curare action, so after an *āsana* position maintained long enough, groups of muscles are "depolarized," that is, completely inert. In other words, through the *āsanas* it is possible to obtain, in an entirely natural way, what medicine has not yet been able to achieve: to induce a selective, curarelike muscular relaxation, limited to particular groups of muscles, without involvement of the entire somatic muscular system, as happens following curare injections. The perfect, selective relaxation induced by the *āsanas* involves a tremendous saving of energy, which is made available for the subsequent stages of the Yogic training, to be redirected inwardly, toward the spinal *Chakras*.

2. When assuming a given position, the disciple is instructed to visualize with closed eyes the somatic structures that are being contracted, until he is able to feel the nervous energy flowing into the contracted muscles. As the training progresses, the disciple learns to expand this feeling and to bring about a visual perception of the autonomous muscles within metameric distribution. In due time, such visual perception becomes actual awareness of the internal organs, felt as areas of heat over the corresponding somatic structures.

The mental concentration focused upon the groups of muscles being contracted and the underlying metamerical visceral structures is a keypoint in the Yogic physical training; without it, the *āsanas* are meaningless.

Long after the position has been released, a deep, segmental muscular relaxation is still maintained, inducing a corresponding "visceral silence" within anatomic boundaries. Through the steady repetition of each *āsana,* every day, morning and evening, the disciple learns gradually to achieve the capability of bringing the body to a total standstill, with the vertebral spine perfectly erect, for prolonged periods of time. The body standstill in turn is essential to quiet down all nervous activities, both on the somatic and on the visceral systems, creating the necessary prerequisites for the subsequent stages of the *Rāja* Yoga path.

3. Each position brings into action all the muscles and all the articulations of a given part of the body. By this method, some somatic muscles usually tending to atrophy because of poor use, such as the muscles of the abdomen, are restored to circulation and good operation.

At the same time, the articulations are subjected to a harmonious effort, unloaded of their burdens, freed from the old "rust," and restored to a good lubrification and to physiological operation. The novice in Yoga training realizes his fact at once when he feels his articulations, already sore and rebellious after the first exercises, rapidly become agile and easily managed as the training progresses. Since medical pathology is well aware of the tremendous importance of a good articular condition, we can easily realize the enormous advantage obtainable through making the articulations soft with the *āsanas.*

4. Each *āsana* position brings into action the vertebral spine, exposing it to tractions, stretchings, and torsions of various degrees. All this prevents and corrects eventual wrong attitudes of the spine in the usual positions, upright, sitting, and lying down. Observe a Yoga disciple, even a novice, and at once you will notice the correct agile and elegant way in which he sits or stands.

5. As you can see from the drawings that follows, the *āsanas* consist of bodily positions that seem to require a great deal of effort. In Yoga training, this effort must be gradually elimi-

nated through a better dynamic and static use of the muscular groups brought into tension by the exercise. An expert Yogi can assume the most difficult positions with an absolutely minimum effort, keeping relaxed whether upright, sitting, or lying down, whether twisting, or directly upside-down, as in the *śīrśāsana*. In other words, he learns to find and keep a position of equilibrium with the best articular action, whatever the position taken by his body.

This ability always to keep in relaxed equilibrium with no effort has an important psychological transposition. The Yogi, through the physical training, gradually learns to keep his psychological equilibrium unaltered, to preserve a perfect psychophysical calm whatever environment position he might happen to find himself in.

Let us now try to analyze in detail a few of the more well-known *āsanas*. This analysis by no means should suggest to the reader that he attempt these "positions" by himself without qualified supervision. *Āsanas*, as all other Yogic techniques, are part of a whole, harmonious psychophysical training, a step in a long path, which should be traveled under the guidance of a true spiritual teacher.

Haṭha Yoga considers this *āsana* the prince of all the *āsanas*, the key position to be assumed during the exercises of *prāṇā-yāma* and the higher steps of *Rāja* Yoga.

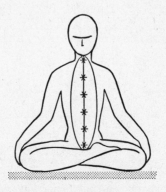

Fig. 1   *Padmāsana*—the "perfect position"

The health advantages of *padmāsana* are to be found in the position of the lower limbs, tightly bent and locked over the hip and knee articulations. By compelling the hip and knee joints to forced flexion, a redistribution of blood circulation is achieved, shifting a larger blood supply from the lower limbs into the abdomen. In consequence, we have an internal blood "transfusion" with increased blood flow through the visceral organs. Modern medicine sometimes tries to achieve similar internal "blood transfusions" by raising the legs of the patients in those emergency situations in which a condition of decreased blood volume is feared.

Moreover, by resting his body solidly on the ground in a triangle formed by the two thighs and by the perineum, with a perfectly perpendicular spine, the Yogi is given a perfect sense of psychosomatic equilibrium. *Padmāsana* is a difficult position; a Westerner who has come to the practice of Yoga in his adult life can seldom keep it for long despite all his good will. Modern Yogic techniques, suited for Caucasians of Western cultures, have substituted for the *padmāsana* a posi-

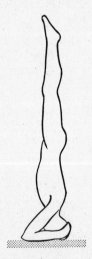

Fig. 2   *Śīrṣāsana*—the "upside-down position"

tion sitting on an armless chair; of *Padmāsana* this latter retains the essential advantages—a perpendicular vertebral spine, a good equilibrium, the lower limbs bent over the hip and knee joints, without the tight leg lock of the original position.

Sīrśāsana is the opposite of and yet of equivalent value to *padmāsana*, a position of perfect upside-down equilibrium, with a solid base of support formed by the triangle—top of the head and forearms with elbows opened at a straight angle. Although seemingly very difficult, with a little training *sīrśāsana* is an exercise that can be performed by whoever is endowed with normal physical health, and allows for an excellent relaxation of all the muscles, since the axis of gravity from the barycenter of the body drops exactly in the supporting triangle.

The physiological advantages are to be found in a greater flow of blood to the head, with a better blood supply to the endocranial nervous centers, and a discharge of blood and weight from the lower limbs. It is an excellent position to subdue circulation ailments of the lower limbs (swellings, varicose veins), or articular lesions, as well as abdominal herniae. The discharge of blood from the bottom to the top influences also the internal organs and partially decongests the kidneys, the bladder, the liver, the intestines, the stomach, and the sexual organs, relieving many ailments from deterioration and poor function of these organs. Obviously, people struck by chronic diseases of the heart and of the vascular system (arteriosclerosis) must avoid *sīrśāsana*. This position, in fact, increases the venous pressure into the right side of the heart, resulting in an improved cardiac output. The increased heart pumping provides for a better distribution of blood to all parts of the body; however, when the heart is in poor condition, an increased venous pressure may end up in pulmonary congestion, edema, and death. Some of the cardiovascular effects produced by *sīrśāsana* have been confirmed through medical investigation upon patients standing in the so-called Trendelenburg position. For surgical purposes, this position is obtained by tilting the operating table, with head down and feet up, at about 30 degrees. Studies on cardiac output and other cardiovascular functions in the Trendelenburg position have indeed confirmed what Yoga claims to be the physiological effects of *śīrṣāsana*.

But *Haṭha* Yoga proposes a further, very important result of the upside-down position, that is, to reverse the direction of the flux of pranic energy. Instead of flowing along the vertebral electric axis, from the positive pole in the skull to the negative pole in the coccyx, that is, from the interior to the exterior, in *śīrṣāsana* the pranic current flows from the negative to the positive pole, from the exterior to the interior. This reversal of current, which is passive in *śīrṣāsana,* will become an act of volition in *prātyahāra* and will allow the Yogi to isolate himself electrically from the external world.

In Sanskrit, *sarva* means "all" and *anga* means "body"; *sarvāṅgāsana* therefore means exercise that summons the whole body to health. Its English translation, "position of the candle," seems to be less appropriate. It is an exercise easily executed by anybody.

The healthy results of *sarvāṅgāsana* are due to a dual mechanism of stretching and isometric contraction on three distinct muscular groups—stretching of the back muscles, contraction

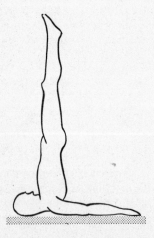

Fig. 3   *Sarvāṅgāsana*—the "position of perfect health"

of the muscles in the abdominal wall, and contraction of the
fore muscles of the neck.

The stretching of the back muscles leads to a reduction of
the basal tension of these muscles, with the elimination of
many muscular stiffnesses resulting from a poor orthopedic
position of the vertebral column. The contraction of the
abdominal muscles restores an often neglected functionality
to them, and at the same time eliminates the fat stored in
the abdominal walls. The visceral muscles, metamerically
corresponding to the lower back and abdominal muscles, are
constituents of all the organs contained in the abdomen. Their
contraction and relaxation, therefore, revitalize in an excellent way the functions of the stomach, the intestines, the liver,
the pancreas, the spleen, the kidneys, the bladder, and of the
uterus in women, eliminating digestive, metabolic, urinary,
and uterine deficiencies and ailments. *Sarvāngāsana* thus leads
to salutary results similar to those obtained from *śīrṣāsana,*
but arrived at through a different mechanism. Moreover,
sarvāngāsana, like *śīrṣāsana,* by decreasing the blood supply to
the pelvic region, helps in time of sexual arousal to gain control over the sex impulses.

And finally, the contraction of the fore muscles of the neck
combined with the pressure of the chin on the chest leads to
a redistribution of the blood in the upper part of the trunk,
with important results. For, while the arterial circulation to
the brain remains normal through the vertebral arteries, the
arterial thrust in the carotids and the venous deflux of the
jugulars are slowed down. Consequently, the thyroid, the thymus (in the young), and the parathyroids receive an increase
in blood flow, which stimulates and improves their function. Modern endocrinology teaches us that the thyroid gland
is a star of the first magnitude in the endocrine constellation,
so much that its deficiency causes cretinism. An improved thyroid function, therefore, is translated into a general well-being
for the entire human organism.

In Sanskrit, *hala* means "plow"; hence; its equivalent in
Western language is the "plow position." The health results
of *halāsana* are analogous to those of *sarvāngāsana* through an
identical mechanism, further stressed on a greater stretching
and a more considerable contraction of the back, abdominal,

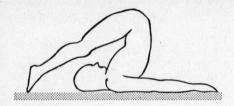

Fig. 4   *Halāsana*—the "extended-arch position"

and neck muscles. By its complete stretching of the vertebral spine, *halāsana* helps to correct many postural defects through the reinforcement of the paravertebral muscles (*see* Appendix); moreover, it may help in relieving some nerve entrapments at the level of the vertebral foramina where the nervous fibers to the back muscles branch off. Finally, like *sarvāngāsana* and *śīrśāsana,* this position shifts the blood flow toward the thoracic and brain regions with similar results upon abdominal, pelvic, and sexual functions. By performing several *halāsanas* in sequence, an alternate pressure upon the chest is obtained, somewhat similar to a cardiac massage, followed by a general benefit upon the cardiovascular function.

Vajrāsana reproduces the tensions and the stretchings of *sarvāngāsana* in reverse order. In fact, here the back muscles are contracted, whereas the abdominal and the neck muscles are stretched considerably. The effects on the visceral muscles are, therefore, of the same kind, and the salutary advantages are complementary to those gained from *sarvāngāsana.* Furthermore, the overturned position, by compelling the knee articulation to a forced flexion, vigorously restores to it its good function. It is a difficult position, very hard to maintain, and should be started in one's early age, before the knees become too "rusty."

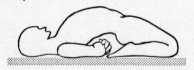

Fig. 5   *Vajrāsana*—the "overturned position"

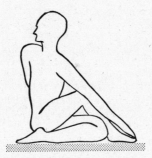

Fig. 6   *Matsyendrāsana*—the "screw position"

This is the only Yoga exercise, with its numerous variations, that requires a maximum torsion of the vertebral column, first on one side, then on the other, causing the vertebrae to rotate one over the other, and to bend, at the same time, to the right or to the left.

The movement of vertebral rotation performs an energetic massage on the motor, sensory, and visceral nervous roots coming out of the spinal cord through the foramina between vertebra and vertebra. The whole somatic and visceral nervous system is thus revitalized. In the forced movements of torsion, the lumbar muscles are especially stimulated to stretch and contract isometrically. This exercise improves considerably the function of the kidneys, metamerically corresponding to the lumbar region. Through a mechanical compression and a better distribution of blood at the lumbar vertebral level, the suprarenal glands are also stimulated. These endocrine glands hold an enormous importance in man's functional economy, so much so that their deficiency is incompatible with life. To revitalize the suprarenal glands means to improve the whole circulatory system, and to promote a "recharge" of energy in the cellular "electric batteries."

In Sanskrit, *mudra* means "symbol," "model"; therefore, this position is intended to be a symbol of Yoga. In fact, it puts

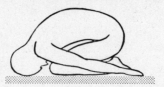

Fig. 7 *Yogamudra*—the "crouched position"

the body in an attitude of inward concentration, which easily transfers to humility. The Yogi in the *Yogamudra* position is a man who has learned to bow before Life and before his Creator.

The analogies of *Yogamudra* are obvious with certain attitudes of religious devotion on the part of the Moslems, traceable also to some forms of adoration in the solemn Catholic rites. Physically, the crouched position is an excellent exercise of tension and of stretching of the back muscles, synergic with other *āsanas* to give the vertebral column back its elasticity.

Our analysis ends here. The seven *āsanas* we have examined constitute the foundations of *Haṭha* Yoga. All the other exercises repeat in some way the fundamental attitudes of these— positions stretched forward, backward, bent to the right or to the left, in torsion, always taking the vertebral spine for their axis of gravity.

When the Yogi has finished his *āsanas* every morning and every evening, and sits relaxed in body and mind for the subsequent stages of his daily mystical practice, he no longer is the normal man that he was before his exercises. He is literally magnetized, charged with bioelectrical energy, activated in the ways I have tried to explain above. The Yogi feels this energy inside himself, in the form of a quiver spreading from the tip of his toes toward his trunk, pervading his internal organs, stopping at his heart, and finally climbing up to a point between the two eyebrows, where it forms a faint luminous point.

The energy patrimony gathered through the *āsanas*, stops here. To illuminate his mind completely, the Yogi needs a superior energy, which cannot come to him from the body. He will call for this energy to come to him from the Cosmos, through the *prāṇāyāma*.

Note For more information about the *āsanas* consult the following
excellent publications:
Muzumdar, S., *The Yogic Exercises* (16)
The "Self-Realization Magazine," published by Self-Realization
    Fellowship, Los Angeles, Calif. (32)

Chapter Five

Energy and
Oxygen Consumption:
A look at
Our Respiration

In the chapter on Nutrition, we spoke of food as the fuel necessary to the human engine, and observed that another element is necessary for the fuel to burn. As everybody knows, the only burning element in the earth's atmosphere is oxygen. Without oxygen, no engine using a process of combustion as its source of energy can function. Many motorists experience this physical truth every day, when the engine of their car has a breakdown because the carburetor is dirty.

Oxygen has to do with a biological cycle strictly connected to the carbon cycle, whose stages are here mentioned in synthesis. From the water in the ground (H_2O = hydrogen + oxygen), oxygen is taken and joined to carbon in the green plants, to form carbohydrates. In the human body, the carbohydrate is divided into its components: hydrogen, oxygen, and carbon. These two last elements are given out in the form of carbon dioxide (CO_2) through lung exhalation. In the atmosphere, carbon dioxide is picked up by the chlorophyll present in the leaves of plants, which separates the carbon from the oxygen, sending the latter back into the atmosphere, to be again used by man through lung inhalation.

It may be worth mentioning here that many concepts dealing with natural phenomena, which are currently accepted by modern biology, actually were first expressed under different semantic terms thousands of years ago, when in the *Vedas* the principle of life was identified with the well-known four elements *air, water, earth, fire,* differently combined one to the other. This conception of Creation was taken up by the Egyptians and worked out in the famous "Doctrine of Hermes." From Egypt, it went to Greece, in the teaching of the philosophers of the School of Miletus: to the four elements, Democritus added a new concept, that of energy, expressed in his theory of the atoms. From Greece, India's most ancient teaching spread to the whole Roman world, reappeared in the alchemy and in the astrology of the Middle Ages, and finally, has emerged again in modern science, which has given an experimental demonstration of it.

But let us go back to man's respiration.

When we speak of respiration, at once we think of the lungs and of their function. In reality, there are two modalities of respiration of which the pulmonary is only one stage, the so-called external respiration. There is a second respiration, called "internal" or of the tissues, which represents the real process of carburetion, or source of life for the organism.

External or Lung Respiration

During lung respiration, man takes in oxygen from the outside atmosphere through his nose, and down the trachea and bronchi he sends it to his lungs where it is passed on to the blood.

We can picture the lung as a big sponge in which a viscous fluid, the blood pumped in by the right side of the heart, circulates continuously.

Just as the sponge is made up of tiny cells, so also the lung consists of innumerable tiny cells called "pulmonary alveoli." Each alveolus is in close touch with the blood current surrounding and permeating it all. Just as a sponge has an elastic stroma that characterizes its elasticity, so also the lung possesses an elastic structure formed by a network of autonomous muscular fibers. This pulmonar elasticity is important in the mechanics of respiration, and an eventual lack of it, from disease or from a poor attitude of the vertebral column, leads to serious respiratory drawbacks, like pulmonary emphysema. In fact, when the chest expands under the action of the respiratory muscles—rib-cage muscles and diaphragm*—the lung dilates and air is sucked in from the atmosphere; during the opposite phase of volumetric reduction of the thorax, the lung also contracts, and ejects the air it contains. In the first stage, called inspiratory, oxygen enters with the air. In the second stage, called expiratory, carbon dioxide goes out with the air. Inspiration and expiration together constitute pulmonary ventilation.

Altogether, the lung has a volumetric capacity of about five liters of air. Of these, only about three liters are ventilated, that is, inhaled and exhaled at each deep respiratory act, whereas a liter to a liter and a half are never ventilated, and stagnate in the lung, totally unused. In physiology, this mass of air stagnating in the lung is called residual volume and evidently constitutes a passivity in the general economy of respiration.

Once it has reached the pulmonary alveoli with the inhaled air, the oxygen is passed on to the blood through the thin walls of the pulmonary alveoli, following partly the hydrodynamic laws, partly the laws of the diffusion of gases. In the blood, it is chemically intercepted by the red corpuscles, which carry it to the tissues. As is well known, oxygen-rich blood circulates in the arteries, whereas the blood full of carbon dioxide flows in the veins. The same laws for the diffusion of the gases regulate the transfer of carbon dioxide from the blood to the lungs, to be exhaled.

Ventilation and circulation are, therefore, the essential elements of external respiration. They are synchronized to each other through a delicate system of nervous control, partly entrusted to the voluntary muscles of respiration, partly to special vegetative reflexes of the heart, of the lungs, and of the arteries. In this way, an increase in ventilation is followed by an increase in circulation, and vice versa. If the two elements

* The diaphragm is a big dome-shaped muscle that separates the thorax from the abdomen. It is considered the chief respiratory muscle of the body.

of respiration are balanced, the condition is called "eupnoea"; when, on the contrary, the two elements go out of phase, the so-called "dispnoea" occurs (the "short breath"), foreshadowing more serious symptoms of respiratory insufficiency, which can quickly become deadly (asphyxy, pulmonary edema, and the like). A breathing suspension is called "apnoea."

The circulation of blood in the lungs is maintained by the heart beats, and is made easier by the movements of inhalation and exhalation. In fact, during inhalation, a negative pressure is produced, promoting the flow of blood from the neck and from the abdomen to the heart, and hence to the lungs. The endopulmonary pressure is reversed and becomes positive during exhalation, thus promoting the expulsion of the blood oxygenated in the lungs. One can easily understand this mechanism by comparing the thorax to a hand holding a sponge immersed in the water: when the hand opens, the sponge expands; when it closes the sponge is squeezed.

In the proposed example, you can observe that if the sponge is kept too long immersed in the water, it becomes so much soaked that it is difficult to squeeze it well. This is what happens in the lungs if one's breath is held during inhalation. In fact, as the negative pressure continues, the lungs become so much soaked with blood that at a certain point, the heart is hardly able to pump more, and increases its pressure which influences the veins of the neck and of the abdomen. Try to hold your breath during inhalation, and after a few seconds, you will observe that the veins of your neck swell up, and you will feel your heart throbbing like mad in your chest, even before the so-called "hunger for air" appears, that is, the necessity to start breathing again.

Many breathing exercises strive to train man to reach apnoea during forced inhalation (chiefly for diving activities): this is a physiological error that can be costly to a man's health. The physiological position of rest for the lungs is that of moderate exhalation, when the refilling of venous blood from the right side of the heart is balanced with the squeezing of oxygenated blood into the left side of the heart. For the untrained man, however, it is almost impossible to hold his breath during exhalation, since the "hunger for air" appears with extreme rapidity, and breathing resumes automatically.

The machines designed for artificial lung ventilation—the so-called "respirators"—try with various devices to adjust continuously the inspiratory and expiratory stages in such a way that the patient may feel comfortable and avoid "fighting the machine," that is, trying to breathe at a different rhythm than the one set by the respirator. The artificial respiratory adjustment is an extremely complicated operation, which further emphasizes how delicate and sophisticated are the physiological mechanisms subserving the vital function of respiration. Rhythms of ventilation cannot be changed easily.

Lung ventilation and circulation require intense activity, that is, expense of energy by the respiratory muscles and by the heart. In the well-balanced individual, this basal waste of energy is moderate, but it can go sky-high, just as soon as a lack of balance results either from illness or from alimentary excesses or from any other kind of excesses in the life of relation. Sometimes, in situations of severe illness, the respiratory activity requires all for itself the energy patrimony produced by the combustions of the organism, which obviously represents a bankruptcy, as if a car used up all the fuel in its tank to make the carburetor work.

It is known that the great sporting champions can display their exceptional performances almost without altering the heart and breathing rhythms. This means that a well-balanced life and a good physical training have taught their heart and lungs to achieve more work without a higher consumption of energy. Just as muscular basal activity is connected to man's mental condition, so too in man's respiratory activity. A harmonious mind matches a rather slow and regular respiration; a troubled psyche speeds up the heart and breathing rhythms. All of us have experienced this occurrence whenever we pant or are short of breath because of some sudden emotion. The statement is reversible: a slow, harmonious, conscious breathing greatly promotes the mental faculties and the relaxation of the mind. This is a matter that characterizes successful men in every field of human activity: no great general on the battlefield, no important industrialist at work, no famous orchestra conductor on the platform, has heart palpitations and difficult breathing before making a decision with an objective mind.

Internal and Tissue Respiration

Through tissue respiration, the oxygen carried by the red corpuscles of the blood is released by the latter to all of the cells making up the tissues of our body. Here, the oxygen is chemically combined with the fuel stored, and ignites the combustion; we have already mentioned one of these combustions when we discussed muscle contraction. The "smoke" of combustion is partly made up of carbon dioxide, which goes to the lungs with the venous blood, and partly by other waste substances, which are eliminated by the kidneys. In Chapter Three, I explained how the production of "smoke" in the combustions of our bodies is connected to the quality of the fuel and to the "draught," that is, the refueling of oxygen. Now we can better understand and specify the close connections existing between respiration and nutrition.

We know that a good draught in a boiler is obtained either by increasing the carburetion, namely the oxygen consumption, or by reducing the flame. The same consideration goes for the human body.

An intense psychophysical activity burns oxygen, that is, requires a high carburetion. But an increased oxygen consumption wants a greater respiratory activity; this means a disproportionate increase of the basal metabolism. Thus a vicious circle of energy waste is caused, similar to the waste we have already seen with regard to the dynamic-specific action of the aliments in a disorderly diet.

In man, this progressive respiratory deficit is usually felt around middle age, when first appears a slight dispnoea caused by strain; that is, one day a man realizes he is short of breath when he climbs certain stairs he used to climb at a nimble run. Then the dispnoea grows worse even without a great effort; later it becomes chronic; hence, other signs of respiratory insufficiency appear, until the heart stops, weary from pumping blood into an exhausted lung. The end is always the same, whether the excess is alimentary, respiratory, or of another nature; and when it comes, most of the time, man realizes he has lived in vain, without ever trying to understand why he had come into the world, toiled, worked, suffered, and now is going to die.

By "lowering the flame" of the metabolic combustion following the standards I have tried to explain in the preceding
chapters, we can reduce the draught. Consequently, the oxygen
consumption and the production of carbon dioxide drop; the
respiratory activity diminishes; the energy patrimony increases
and the whole health of the body improves surprisingly.

Human respiration can be synthetically expressed in this
way, following the pattern of figurative expression that has
already been used many times before in this book. During
external respiration, the somatic man, through his respiratory
work with a voluntary character, breathes for his vegetative
brother to whom he yields the fruit of his continuous labor,
oxygen. The vegetative man has but an indirect control over pulmonary respiration, through the heart, lung, and artery reflexes.
In return, during internal respiration, he works for himself
and his two "brothers," yielding bioelectric energy for the life
of relation and for the production of hormones.

Breathing, therefore, represents a deep connection of the
three parts making up the human entity, one with another.
The metameric organization of the body makes the somatic
man and his vegetative brother solid in their muscular activity,
but only breathing keeps the three "men" of the human
trinity united into One, even though unconsciously, since all
three depend on respiration for the transformation of vital
energy that is the foundation of their life. Control of breathing, therefore, can be one important tool to restore the three
separate parts into a Conscious Unit.

But breathing is still something more. In fact, it represents
man's most direct link with his environment. Lights, sounds,
colors, and odors can give us information about the world
surrounding us, but none of these sensations has a direct grasp
on us. In fact, each of these sensations must be transformed
into perception before it can be changed into conscious
knowledge, and we know that perception works according to
entirely individual psychological patterns: a symphony by
Mozart can appear wonderful to one man, and most boring to
his neighbor.

On the other hand, breathing has an immediate grasp on
every man. The inhaled oxygen goes directly to the tissues

without any individual elaboration, and here "carburizes" the organism according to chemical reactions, similar for all of creation. Identical is the process of combustion in a man's muscle and in the explosion of a volcano—there are quantitative, not qualitative, differences. Oxygen does not have a "sensitive, perceptive, and reactive individuality." Reduce the oxygen in a room, and all those who are shut in there will react in the same way, with minimum subjective differences.

What do we breathe? If I open a textbook of physiology, I I find that man breathes atmospheric air, which is made up of about 20 percent oxygen and 70 percent nitrogen, the rest being various other gases. These figures are correct, but they are not all. In the air we breathe there are, besides oxygen, nitrogen, and helium, lights, sounds, colors, ultra-violet and ultra-red rays, ultra-sounds, Alpha, Beta, Gamma rays, and so on. In the atmosphere, there is an infinite variety of electromagnetic vibrations operating at different wave lengths. Some of these, very few, affect our sense organs, whereas the majority are lost to us unless we resort to special devices, such as radio, television, radar, and the like.

The electromagnetic waves pierce the atmosphere, but they do not belong to the atmosphere. They are manifestations of a single energy—cosmic energy, the Hindus' *Prana,* that still somewhat mysterious entity which the Cosmos is made of, which in modern physics represents the only concept of the Absolute. For, in our world of relativity, the speed of light, vibratory manifestation of the Cosmos, is the only absolute datum beyond which the human mind cannot go (*Fiat lux—* it is written in Genesis—*et lux facta est*).

In his philogenetic immaturity, still lost behind the delusions of *tamas,* man cannot yet perceive by direct intuition the marvels of Creation in the air he breathes. The "Music of the Stars" and the "Light of the Celestial Spheres" are barred to him. In a literal sense, "he has eyes, and does not see; he has ears, and does not hear." He lives in an earthly paradise of fragrances, lights, colors, sounds, harmonious radiations, and only with difficulty can he perceive some of them through his material senses and through the rudimentary radio, television, and electronic sets. Caught by the immoderate desire to live on the material level, man has transformed the divine Act of Inhalation* into a breathless search for oxygen, which allows him to "burn" better, to "burn" quicker, to "burn" all, until in the end he realizes he has burnt out himself and the Divine Gift he had received.†

To climb back up, it is necessary to reverse the spiral process, to start to "burn less." *Yama* and *niyama* partially provide for this goal with their careful and wise rules of nutritional, mental, and moral hygiene. The *āsanas* offer further help, teaching how to produce more energy with less burning and waste. *Prāṇāyāma* finally completes the cosmic rehabilitation, teaching how to "master the *prāṇa*." In its Sanskrit semantic, in fact, *prāṇāyāma* means "control of the *prāṇa*" through various techniques connected with respiration. In our language, we could roughly call *prāṇāyāma* "voluntary controlled respiration," using a definition borrowed from contemporary medicine.

In order to understand *prāṇāyāma* as one of the key-points in Yogic training, we should first understand well the meaning of the *prāṇa* concept in Hindu thought and in the philosophy behind it. *Prāṇa* is an omnipotent force that moves the entire Universe. Man himself is immersed in *prāṇa* according to the three modalities of *tamas, rajas,* and *satvas*. At the present stage of evolution, man is little aware of the pranic (cosmic) forces, and consequently heavily identifies himself with matter, deluding himself in thinking that *he is a body*. Man also forgets that matter is nothing else but condensed energy in continuous transformation. Accepting life at a material level, he must therefore accept the laws of matter's continuous deterioration, decay, and change. However, the ontological spark of Divine Intelligence, which is man's essence, keeps suggesting

---

* And the Lord God formed man from the mud of the earth and inhaled in his face the breath of Life, and man became a living creature, 'made' in his Creator's own image and likeness" (Gen. 1:24, 2:7).

† Conceptual association between "fire and burning" and "hell" is common to many formal religious doctrines. The same concepts, probably through the Sanskrit roots of our words, have entered our language, expressing themselves in statements such as: "I have a burning desire," "he is burning with hate or lust," and the like.

to him that "Joy" is a divine heritage, uniquely reserved to the
dignity of man.

Unfortunately, man usually misunderstands the Divine
Whisper calling for Cosmic Joy, and confuses it with the heavy
pleasures of the body. As a consequence, he wastes vital energy
(which is also a particular form of *prāṇa*) to feed his senses
with a variety of stimulations, born out of an unending chain
of material desires. The more he dwells on matter, the more
he needs "fleshly" nutrition to keep himself alive, and the
more he will "burn." The more he "burns" out oxygen, the
less he can "feel" the *prāṇa* on which he lives. The less he
feels the pranic forces within himself, the more he sinks into
matter, floating his "island of consciousness" with heavy mate-
rial- oriented contents.

The concept of *karma* has already been mentioned along
the course of this book; we may now understand it better in
connection with what has been said concerning the *prāṇa*. The
"Law of *Karma*," or the "Law of Cosmic Causation," is the
moral law of the Universe; it states that the effects of our
actions must be experienced by the individual who has performed them. In its deep value, the Law of *Karma* outlines the
fact that there is a Divine, intelligent plan of Creation where
everything in nature, as well as among humans, is conditioned
and dependent upon something else that has preceded it, in
an ordered relationship of cause and effect. Being a moral law,
karma is also binding, in the sense that we cannot reap fruits
of actions better than the actions themselves. If we steal in
order to gain happiness for us, we delude ourselves badly,
because sooner or later the rebounding effect of the stealing
shall hit us back, stealing something away from us, be it our
freedom because of imprisonment, our own health, or some
dear one's, and so on.

The desire for the fruits of our actions, through the interplay of pranic forces, is the binding link between what we are,
what we strive to be, and what we have actually been in the
past. The concept of *karma* may be better understood if we
think of ourselves as swimming in the great ocean of the
prāṇa. If we set in motion big waves, then by the same big
waves we shall be hit, *unless we learn how to get out of the
ocean* (*see* also Diagram C). *Prāṇāyāma* is one effective way to

rise above the "pranic ocean" and gain "freedom in action," that is, freedom to behave outside the binding karmic forces of cause and effect, as I have tried to explain in the diagram at the end of this chapter.

In the *Bhagavad-Gita*, the Lord-Krishna describes *prāṇā-yāma* in this way: "By exposing his inhaling breath to the action of his exhaling breath, and his exhaling breath to the action of his inhaling breath, the Yogi neutralizes both. In this way, he achieves the cosmic energy in his heart, and brings it under his control." Inside this obscure definition of the *Bhagavad-Gita* is hidden a treasure of wisdom that medicine has just started to discover and to apply. Let's try to analyze it, if only it is possible to translate into words; an experience like *prāṇāyāma* should be lived instead of being described.

A healthy ventilation of the lungs is attained when the following prerequisites are achieved: (1) an erect position of the vertebral column, with the rib cage held in a relaxed upright position, so as to avoid compressions upon the lungs and the other organs (heart and great vessels) contained in the thorax; (2) a deep, slow inhalation, first using the diaphragm as a suckering pump, and then expanding the rib cage with the help of the intercostal and other muscles of the thorax; (3) a slow exhalation, using mostly the diaphragm in reverse action as squeezing pump; (4) a regular breathing rhythm, so that the exhaling period is slightly longer than the inhaling phase; for instance, if you inhale for three seconds, you should exhale for five; (5) a regular ventilatory rest after exhalation; this rest phase should be at least equal to the inhaling period—three seconds of inhalation to five seconds of exhalation to three seconds of rest in exhalation.

Following a regular, slow, and deep breathing, the oxygenation of the blood is known to improve consistently; in consequence, the internal respiration also improves. In other words, regular, harmonious breathing rhythms do improve our tissue carburetion.

However, few of us are capable of breathing in a really harmonious way. Our voluntary control over the respiratory movements is quite limited, being mostly governed by unhealthy habits of living. You just try to follow the above-mentioned breathing rhythm for a little while, and most

likely you will soon feel an unpleasant hunger for air which
will force you, in a reflex way, to resume your habitual rhythm
of respiration.

Basically, *prāṇāyāma* consists of a number of techniques
aimed at changing the inhaling and exhaling rhythms of ventilation into harmonious sequences under the control of will
power, without triggering unpleasant sensations. The exhaling
period is gradually increased following deep and slow inhalation, while the respiratory rest is extended in proper proportion. In time, the ventilation rate becomes very slow—around
4 to 6 per minute in a trained Yogi—perfectly regular, with
frequent periods of prolonged expiratory apnoea. This consciously induced expiratory arrest is experienced as a feeling
of extreme peace in the mind and in the body, with no air
hunger whatsoever.

At this point, probably, a biological cycle in progressive
improvement has begun, which would explain the prolonged
and pleasant apnoea in exhalation. A perfect oxygenation
insures an almost drossless combustion, therefore reduces the
work of the liver and of the kidneys. There is less carbon
dioxide to be eliminated. But also the oxygen refueling tends
to diminish, because of a smaller demand by the tissues. The
breathing rhythms are proportionately reduced, until breathing, spontaneously and without effort, stops. In turn the heart,
having less dross to "sweep out" of the tissues and send to the
liver and to the kidneys, can finally allow itself a little rest,
and consequently reduces its work. The rhythm of the heart
beat is reduced along with the reduction of breathing, and
almost stops. In a trained Yogi, the pulse can drop from the
70 beats per minute which are normal, down to 40 to 30 beats
per minute during the practice of *Prāṇāyāma*. The physical
sensation of the "silence of the heart" is wonderful in its
relaxing equivalence and cannot be described.

Again it must be stressed that *prāṇāyāma*, without the
preparatory stages of *yama, niyama,* and the regular practice
of *āsanas,* is meaningless and useless. The "cosmic rehabilitation"—of which *Prāṇāyāma* is a key point—must first start in
the heart of the disciple and be demonstrated in his commitment to moral living. Altogether, the rules of *yama* and *niyama*
are capable of producing a great deal of reduction in the endless chain of desires, which usually feed our daily activities.

Along with the *āsanas,* they are contributory in producing mental and physical states of rest, with greatly reduced bodily combustions.

Prāṇāyāma is a time-honored, highly sophisticated practice, which should be approached with proper care for all details, wisely following the directions given by the Spiritual Teacher. To sit for *Prāṇāyāma* with a stomach full of meaty food, with a mind filled with contrasting desires, like monkeys in a cage, with no spiritual commitment, would be like sailing the ocean with no knowledge of the art of navigation, going nowhere, if not ending up among the rocks.

As the Yogi learns to control the *prāṇa* through voluntary attentive breathing, he becomes progressively aware of the cosmic energy entering his lungs with the inhaled air. It is sometimes perceived as air rich in ozone, as if he were on top of a high mountain, so to speak. The example is quite appropriate, since we know from physics that ozone is produced when high energy radiation from the sun strikes the oxygen in the earth's atmosphere. The Yogi feels this luminous cosmic energy come down in his lungs, transfer into his blood, and make for his body organs.

With a long training, the Yogi acquires the ability to guide the consciously absorbed pranic energy to his internal organs, being able to perceive selectively each part of them. This is not pure imagination or auto-suggestion, but an objective fact. You can yourself get an idea of it if you try to concentrate all the power of your attention on the fingers of one hand held at the level of your shoulder. After a few minutes of mental strain, you will probably perceive a slight tingling at the tip of your fingers, which will leave you a little surprised. Multiply that perception by a hundred thousand, and you will have an idea of what the Yogi feels during the conscious taking possession of his body.

One medical explanation for your tingling and for the Yogi's power over the organs of the human body lies in the relationship between mental states and vascular functions. When you blush or turn pale because of an emotion, you do nothing but unconsciously transmit the echo of your psychological attitude to the arteries of your face. With *prāṇāyāma,* the Yogi has transformed this unconscious reflex into conscious will, and can therefore shift the flow of his circulation in the different parts of his organism, thus stimulating or reducing their functional potentials. Just as you perceive a sensation of heat when you blush, so the Yogi perceives an identical sensation of heat when, in his mind, he visualizes his liver or his heart, as he leads the pranic current to them. In due time, the disciple is then instructed on how to consciously guide the pranic current to the spinal cord, greatly raising the electrical charge in the *Chakras*. Each one of them consequently becomes like a magnet capable of attracting to itself the bioelectrical energy diffused throughout the body. After prolonged practice, the Yogi actually feels this concentrated energy along his spinal cord like a humming tune, and is ready to channel it up, merging into Cosmic Consciousness.

In this way, day and night, month after month, year after year, the three separate parts of the human body are bound together under the control of Consciousness and Will Power. No longer do three men exist, but a single Superman, or rather, indeed a True Man was born.

At this stage of evolution, the Yogi really knows he is immersed in the infinite Ocean of Cosmic Energy, himself a part of the Universe. Not only does he perceive the *prāṇa* in the air he breathes, but likewise he feels its presence in the vegetables, in the fruit, in the cereals he feeds on, he smells it in the scent of the flowers, hears it in the sounds, sees it in the lights and in the colors that make this earthly world of ours so beautiful to those who can see it correctly. In other words, the Yogi has inserted his own vital cycle into Nature's biological cycles, and feels one with the whole Creation. Carbon, oxygen, nitrogen, hydrogen, and the other chemical elements of which our body is made up, are the same ones present in the sun, in the planets, in the stars. From this intuitive solidarity, the Yogi comes to love all of Creation, and starts to realize the Unity that lies behind the various phenomena. St. Francis of Assisi, in his beautiful *Canticle of Creatures,* has left us a delicate poetic interpretation of this Universal Intuition when he calls the moon and the stars, the wind, the water, the fire, the earth, and the corporeal death, by the name of "brother" and "sister."

Since India has achieved independence, there has been a

renewed interest in the scientific investigation of Yoga practices. A committee of scientists was charged years ago to investigate the healing activities in a number of Yoga Centers
throughout India. Two medical institutions in particular have
devoted themselves to the scientific study of Yoga. They are
the Kivalyadhama Institute of Lonavala and the Yoga Institute of Bombay, with some marginal researches made at the
All-India Institute of Medical Sciences in New Delhi. In the
United States, also, a few research projects have been designed
to investigate the fascinating mysteries of Yoga from a scientific standpoint. I will try here briefly to outline for the general public some of the data from such research, directly
quoting from medical journals.

1. The results of the committee investigation about the
healing effects of Yogic practices have been disappointing
from the standpoint of objective medical evidence. In its
conclusions, the same committee has pointed out that, as
Yoga is not a religious denomination, neither is it a medical
specialty. It is a spiritual path to attain God-Communion.
As such, Yogic āshrams do not keep records of patients
according to the standards of the medical profession. Healing of body disharmonies and disfunctions is viewed as a
natural consequence of the training, and not too much
attention is paid to it. The Yogi is pragmatically interested
in hygienic as well as in moral laws; both must be respec·ed
as a price to pay and as a reward to enjoy on the way to
Spiritual Illumination. He pays due respect to the health of
the body as to all life manifestations, but is not hypo-
chrondriac about it.

*(Ministry of Education, India: Report of the Committee
on Evaluation of Therapeutical Claims of Yogic Practices, 1964).*

2. Electrocardiographic and electroencephalographic re-
cordings of Yogis after prolonged *prāṇāyāma* have shown
normal waking patterns.*

(E.E.G. and Clinical Neurophysiology, 1961).

* The *electroencephalogram* is a recording of the electrical activities of
the brain, as they are shown in different patterns, during waking periods,
sleep, and other normal and abnormal brain functions.

3. The electrical resistance of the skin is raised after pro-
longed *prāṇāyāma*.†
*(E.E.G. and Clinical Neurophysiology, 1957, Journal of
Neuropsychiatry, 1963).*

4. The average oxygen consumption in the body of a Yogi
who was sealed in an air-tight box for two subsequent periods of time—eight hours the first time and ten the second—
was found greatly reduced during the period of observation;
the carbon dioxide output from the lung also decreased
during the same period of time. Even when breathing air in
which the oxygen content had been reduced and the carbon
dioxide increased was pumped into the box, the Yogi did
not change his ventilatory rhythm, as all of us would have
been forced to do.
(Indian Journal of Medical Researches, 1961).

Pending further evidence, the above researches and others
along the same line of investigation seem to demonstrate
that the practice of *prāṇāyāma* induces a deep relaxation
both in the muscular structures and in the vegetative nervous system, without drowsiness or sleep.
(American Journal of Psychotherapy, 1963).

With *prāṇāyāma* all medical investigations must stop at
least at our present capability. The final ascents of Yoga are
no longer susceptible of medical analysis. They are subjective
experiences that must be lived to be understood, and cannot
be analyzed. At the present stage of human evolution, health
sciences are and must be necessarily concerned mainly with
average human beings, afflicted as we are by all the diseases
born out of and fed by our psychophysiological disharmonies.
Those who wish to expand their ideas of higher Yoga steps
and its mystical experiences are advised to read *Autobiography
of a Yogi*, by Paramahansa Yogananda, one of the finest and
truly inspiring books ever written for the West on Yoga.

---

† The *Electrical Skin Resistance Test* is one of the most sensitive methods to demonstrate changes of activity in the sympathetic nervous system.
The electrical resistance of the skin is raised in the absence of emotional
excitement, during deep muscular relaxation, and after the intake of drugs
that inhibit the function of the sympathetic system.

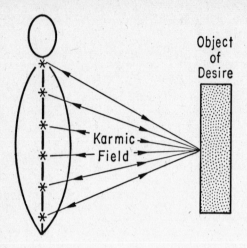

Reinforcing the karmic field

DIAGRAM C When we perform an action in response to a desire, the waves of energy triggered by it hit the object of our desire and rebound back to us. With repeated "back-firing," one or more of our *Chakras* will soon become involved in the rebounding waves and consequently it will become bound to the object, as if magnetically attracted to it. The links between ourselves and the desired object will be compounded according to the number of the *Chakras* involved, each one reinforcing the Karmic field. The end-result is that we have lost our freedom so far as that particular object is concerned, because we are conditioned by it. We express this slavery in affirmations such as "I want it with all my heart," "I feel it in my stomach," "It moves my heart," and so on.

Contemporary medicine is well aware of these phenomena. They have been identified and investigated as emotional expressions, sustained mainly through the activity of the sympathetic system (see Chapter One).

Learning how to gain control of the *Chakras* through *prāṇāyāma* and *pratyāhāra,* the Yogi is actually capable of permanently breaking the links with all objects of desire, and merge free in Cosmic Consciousness.

Part Two

Some Common
Human Problems:
From the
Perspective
of Yogic
Philosophy

Chapter Six

Sex-Energy: The Sexual Problems in the Light of Yoga

Sex is one of the most diffuse arguments of our time, one of the problems most debated by the public opinion, and one of the favorite subjects of literature, theater, and film productions.

Actually, the so-called "problem of sex" is a human artefact. It reflects the anxieties of humans to cover under various labels the wrong exercise of a natural instinct, such as the instinct of reproduction is.

Freud is often misquoted to be the father and the founder of the so-called "sex psychology." Actually, he was only the expression of an age of romantic pessimism, tainted with materialism, coming down from Schopenhauer to Nietzsche, through Hegel and Karl Marx. Sigmund Freud stands like a giant in the history of modern psychology, and I dare to say that many are those who quote him without having ever made an effort to understand his ideas.

It is true that Freud emphasized the importance of sex in human behavior, but he also said that "in a normal sex life, no neurosis is possible." This statement comes as close to the Yoga point of view as few others do in contemporary sciences. Indeed, neurotic behaviors do not stem from a normal sex reason, but from repressed sexual desires and fantasies, which are perversions of sex. When some of our contemporary writers and thinkers use the name of Freud to feed us with all kinds of erotic fantasies and sexual details, they are as much distorting his ideas as Hitler mistook the ideas of Hegel, and as some "leftists" of today misunderstand Karl Marx. So far as the human personality is viewed only from a strictly biological standpoint, the psychological and spiritual sides of every problem do not make much sense. However, shut out of the main door, these forces do come back through the back door, go in hiding in the unconscious well, and generate inner tensions.

The greatest insult one can do to man is to compare him to an animal, blindly controlled by unconscious instincts. Even though up to a certain point life's biological laws are similar for man and animal, man's nervous system has a much greater complexity than that of his closest relative on the biological scale, the ape. There is, moreover, a fundamental difference between man and animal: Man has the capability to reason, animals do not. The human being might degenerate down to a level lower than the animal (no tiger has ever let millions of other tigers die in a concentration camp, for the sheer pleasure of making them suffer), but as a whole he cannot be compared to an animal. Nature's primeval instincts of reproduction and self-preservation exist also in man, but they are subjected to the control of man's psychological functions. Man's sexual behavior, therefore, is not a true product of the instinct, but the result of an interpretation of the instinct on the part of the mind, in terms of learned habits, emotions, and cognitive processes.

In Chapter Two, I tried to explain "consciousness" and "unconscious" and the relationship between the two. Some Freudians seem to think that only the unconscious prevails in the sexual life, whereas some superficial moralists suppose that only the conscience speaks, without showing how it could be developed.

On the other hand, man's behavior, and not only in the sexual field, is the balance between actions dictated by the conscious mind and actions controlled by unconscious forces. For this reason, I dare to state there is no sexual problem per se, but only a particular modality of man's behavior in the course of his earthly life.

To understand the role of sex, we must extend our discussion a little, and examine separately the two terms of the equation shown above: sexual instinct as a biological factor, and its psychological interpretation.

Biological Factor

In Nature, the chief purpose toward which all the living organisms aim is the preservation of the species. In the animal world, the individual is the fleeting instrument of the lasting species, the mortal remains designed to preserve and to protect the potentially immortal germinative element. In Nature, the individual has no importance, and all the numerous and complicated mechanisms brought into action to preserve his life aim at warranting the survival of the species.

The generated organism is the product of partitions of a single cell from the generating organism, that is, of the fertilized egg. Upon receiving the male element, the egg undergoes numerous divisions and subdivisions, until it will give birth to the hundred quadrillion cells of which the human body is made up.

As is well known, the egg is prepared in the ovary where maturation readies it for infiltration by the male element. The ovary produces hormones important for preparing the uterus to receive the fertilized egg. If fertilization does not occur, the unused egg is ejected from the ovary which secretes another hormone to bring the uterus back to its pre-existing condition. In the woman there are, therefore, two possible cycles of hormone activity. One cycle, called the fertilizing cycle, starts with the maturation of the egg, specializes with the preparation of the uterus, and ends with the fertilization of the egg. Once the fertilization is achieved, new hormones are provided to support the product of the conception until the birth of the new organism, and to feed it during the first months of its life outside the uterus. The second possible female cycle, called the asexual cycle, starts and continues like the former, with the difference that the uterus, because of nonfertilization, at a certain point degenerates into that secretion known by the term *menstruation*.

In Chapter Three, I mentioned the relationship existing between nutrition and reproduction, pointing out that the material metabolism provides not only for the energetic necessities of the individual, but also for the needs of the species, transforming the alimentary energy into sexual energy. Here I want to clarify this concept in further detail.

Two forms of biological energy are needed for the reproductive function: a sexual energy, supplied by the male and female hormones, produced by the ovary and by the testicle out of energetic material coming from the foods, and a reproductive energy, which is characteristic of the spermatozoon and of the egg. The two male and female elements originate from identical embryological structures, and are endowed with a reproductive potentiality that cannot be restored through food intake. It constitutes an energetic patrimony, which the human being—like the animal—carries within himself from birth, and that cannot be changed by the human will. Its exhaustion, as everybody knows, involves profound changes in the woman and to a lesser extent in a man, known as the climacteric.

We can synthesize the aforesaid notions in the following way. In every being living on earth two biological entities co-exist: an individual entity and an ontological collective entity, that is, the species, present in the individual in the form of an egg or of a spermatozoon. The individual supplies the organs of the species with the (sexual) energy needed to make their reproductive potentiality actual, the species makes its necessities felt by the individual according to ancestral modalities and collective archetypes: the voice of the species in the individual is called sexual instinct or instinct of reproduction. It follows that "to obey one's sexual instinct" in Nature means "to listen to the voice of one's species," and therefore, to procreate other individuals in order to transmit the life of the species. Every animal listens to this voice and exercises its sexual rights, procreating. Man does not: he wants to exercise a natural right, but evade the duties inherent to the exercised right. Man alone, in all Nature, resorts to antifecundity devices!

As one can see, to compare distorted sexual behaviors in humans to animal sex activities on the ground that both men and animals follow their instincts is basically wrong. If there is a field where man does not obey the instinct, that is, the voice of the human species, it is in his sexual activities.

Psychological Factors

In humans, the psychological sexual life is governed by two main forces: one force that we could call "love" (with the small "l," not to be confused with the true meaning of "Love," as we shall see further on), and another that we could identify as the force of habits. The "force of love" drives us into the desire to give ourselves to someone else, while habits govern the modalities of this giving. According to the particular personality of each one of us, different situations can be pictured: (1) a rational sexuality, where the drive for love is matched against concepts of right-wrong, acceptable-unacceptable; (2) an emotional sexuality, where we "love" according to an evaluation in terms of like-dislike, pleasant-unpleasant; (3) a sensual sexuality, where the only evaluation is directed toward feeding the senses with ever-new sexual stimulations, outside any drive for "love," that is, sexual behavior is exclusively ego-centered, with no wish to give, but only to achieve self-gratification.

It is obvious that the first modality leads to social and ethical relations that are expressed within the institution of marriage: in them the voice of the human species finds the best conditions to make itself heard. The second modality, when constantly prevalent, may lead to immoderate sexual behaviors, outside the socioethical order, often suffering deep distortions in contrast with the interest of the species. The myth of Don Juan symbolizes this psychological attitude, eternally in search of a sexual ideal, in endless changes. Today psychology recognizes that such a highly emotional sexual behavior is often the manifestation of immature personalities seeking integration and reassurance through the exercise of sex. The third psychosexual modality is the most immoderate of all and the farthest from the laws of nature: the phenomenon of prostitution feeds on it. The sexual activity is aimed at the only end of material pleasure, and constitutes the most serious deprivation of the instinct. But the violated Nature takes a hard revenge and transforms the sexual system into a parasite of the entire organism. Man thus starts a descending spiral among the most dangerous and the most dramatic: the desire for sexual satisfaction through the pleasure of the senses is soon transformed into sex lust, that is, into a mental activity all turned to the pleasures of sex. All of the body's sensory stimuli and the mental functions become enslaved to this end. The waste of energy increases, the alimentary needs rise immoderately, gluttony appears, which turns into hypernutrition to supply extra energy at the request of the sexual parasite, and so on.

At their extreme, situations of habitual sexual disharmonies may eventually merge into overt sociopathic traits. Our contemporary Western culture, by feeding our curiosity about sex with a variety of erotic fantasies and pseudoscientific information, seems to push our behavior toward ever more distorted sensory-sexual expressions.

The psychosexual modalities outlined characterize the sexual behavior of a human being, but do not represent a constant function of the mind. They can always change one into the other, with a tendency to involution rather than to evolution. It is always possible that a marriage born under the sign of feeling will degenerate into a sensual-sexual relation between husband and wife, with a total disdain for the instinct, or is wrecked in extramarital relationships of the same kind. Newspapers, courtrooms, and physicians' waiting rooms are full of the painful echoes of these sexual involutions.

In Nature, the instinct of reproduction is not exhausted in the sexual act of mating, but is extended to the period of the suckling of the progeny, transforming itself into a "maternal or paternal instinct of the animal." As soon as the progeny has become self-sufficient, the obligations to the species are fulfilled, and the animal resumes its individual liberty, ready to answer the next sexual call with his mate.

In human society, the institution of the family substitutes for the instinct, and is centered around the couple whose progeny is but its natural product. Therefore, it is not dissolved when the children have grown up, but should last until one of the two consorts dies. In the social and moral human cultures, the family should represent the experimental training ground where man and woman can find the most favorable conditions for their progressive psychological maturation, helping each other in the hard work of bringing into light the dark areas of their respective personalities, interpreting and transmitting their experiences to their offspring.

The sanctity of marriage, which is a common concept in all great religious systems in the world, is based upon the assumption that man and woman have been united in wedlock according to a "God's Will," meaning the play of Karmic forces of Cosmic Causation. These same moral forces support the mutual efforts of the couple in order to help each other toward ever-expanding spiritual experiences throughout life, while at the same time discharging their duties toward the human species within the ethical codes of society. Consequently, to break the wedlock is similar to going against the cosmic forces of *Karma* that determined the meeting of the two mates. In doing so, the individual takes changes of generating more troubles than he wants to solve with the dissolution of his marriage.

It is not the task of this book to probe the psychology of the family, but to frame the problem and examine alternative ways to deal with it.

Schematically, we can say that the psychological situation that has characterized the mating is projected on to the family. If this mating has been the product of a conscious loving feeling, the family structure will be solid and the children well bred, but if the husband and the wife have been led to mate by mixed feelings supported by a prevailing sensual desire, they will see in their children almost an accident of their pleasure and a future obstacle.

There are profound differences between man's paternal or maternal instinct and its equivalent in the animal. For the animal, the instinct is obedience to the voice of the species, whereas in the human it is the expression of one's individual ego. Parents often tend to see themselves in their children, with a process of identification that will be the more marked the more their own personalities are maladjusted. This is love with the small "l," the "love" which is expressed in a selfish function: I love my children because they are mine, I love my wife or my husband because she or he is mine, I love my family, my society, my country because they are property that belongs to me or is useful to me. All is made relative to our little personality, which represents only a dim light in the potential illumination of our whole Being.

We know, in fact, that "I" and "my" refer to a single, small part of our ontological entity. To relate everything to our little "ego" means to distort the world, to make life wretched, to cripple the whole of Creation. How many fathers and mothers destroy their children by transferring onto them their frustrations, spurring them on to ways unsuited for them, but which the parents would have wanted to follow themselves, in the pursuit of some obscure ambitions or passions? Who can measure the sum of unhappiness, crimes, domestic "feuds" and wars, accumulated in the course of the centuries because of the wrong identification of the individual ego in the family?*

The establishment of the couple in marriage and the institution of the family, cell of the social life, hold a fundamental importance in the human society. For this reason, society has never abandoned it to the individual initiative, but ever since the most remote civilizations has made it the object of a civil code, within the framework of social and moral laws. But the social standards regarding sex reflect collective interests and neglect those of the individual. Provided that the "social façade" is clean, Western cultures do not care much about the miseries and the tensions of each man, who is usually abandoned to himself in a riddle of contrasting instincts and habits.

Psychology and psychiatry try to cope with a variety of sexual and marital problems and are often successful in offering some help and some behavioral manipulation. However, they necessarily must approach each problem from the outside, using methods that must be interpreted and accepted by the individual in order to be effective. But the mind works with the power it possesses, and cannot consent to outside education, except within the limits it understands and which comply

---

* ". . . I have come to separate the son from the father, the daughter from the mother, the daughter-in-law from the mother-in-law; and man's enemies will be those of his household. He who loves his father and mother more than he loves me, is not worthy of me; and he who loves his son and daughter more than he loves me, is not worthy of me. . . ." (Matt. 10:35-37).

with it. It is like a circumlocution: Psychology wants to enlighten the dark areas of the mind, but man's psyche can understand only the educational teaching inside the limits within which it has already been enlightened.

For example, a sensual man understands and accepts the relationships between sex and nutrition with great difficulty. In his zeal to control sex, he will take comfort in greater eating, and will never be able to get rid of his sexual slavery. Fatally, one day he will grow weary and will start thinking there are errors in what he has been taught. Then he will speak of uncontrollable sexual impulses, of man's right to the pleasure of the sense, or of desperation, according to whether he is an extrovert or an introvert.

If the sexual problem in humans is the manifestation of a basic distortion of a natural instinct, sustained by a high-frequency emotional discharge, it is obvious that the solution of the problem lies mainly in restoring the sex instinct to its natural function, while bringing the emotional components under an intelligent, volitional control. I think that Yogic training is one of the most effective disciplines, capable to achieve the above-mentioned goals within a comprehensive approach.

At the beginning of this chapter, I have said that the sexual instinct is the Voice of the Species speaking in the individual. Hindu philosophy completes and transfers this concept to a universal level, stating that the sexual instinct is a means by which the "Word" of the Creator reaches the individual through the species.*

---

* This conception is found at the basis of all pseudoreligious cults that propose to revive the Divine Voice in man through ritual sexual exercise. The orgiastic cults of certain ancient Mediterranean and Oriental divinities, in their obvious degeneration, had, however, at their basis a longing for God. In the same way would work the haunting rhythm of the sacred dances of certain African tribes of today, with a clearly sexual content. When our youths fidget in the frenzy of certain black rhythms, they certainly do not even imagine they are "miming" something that originally was intended to be "sacred." Still today, in India lives an ancient doctrine with a religious-sexual background, called *tantras,* whose interpretation is especially obscure and difficult to us Westerners.

Yoga compares the species to a great river flowing from its source to the ocean. Source and ocean are one, that is, Spirit. Individual lives are like canals flowing from the river into the fields of the earth to irrigate them. The water of the canals comes back to the river and from here to the ocean through different paths in a slow and meandering way. Through ignorance (*avidyā*), man has lost his consciousness of the river whence he originates, and identifies himself with the earth on which flows that slender trickle of water that is his individual life, separated from the power of the river. Ridding him of his ignorance, he will come back to the river without effort, just as the water in the canals comes back to the river naturally, as soon as it has been rid of its soil debris.†

The "river power" of the species, that is, the reproductive energy in man, lies collected at the base of the spinal cord, in a *Chakra* called *mūlādhāra* (in Sanskrit, mula means "root"; mūlādhāra is the root joining the individual to the species).

We recall that mūlādhāra corresponds approximately to the sacral plexus of human anatomy, where the nervous centers controlling the genital functions are situated.

Hindu symbolism calls the genital force *kuṇḍalinī*, and compares it to a serpent rolled up at the end of the vertebral column. When the serpent is too much solicited toward the outside, because of an immoderate sexual activity, it offers the apple of sensual illusion (*māyā*), which enchains man to the wrong egocentric identification with matter. On the other hand, if man learns to control *kuṇḍalinī*, then the serpent unrolls upward and climbs inside the vertebral column, until

† A Yoga experience in the deep stages of meditation subjectively confirms this Hindu conception. The first contact of the Yogi with Pranic Energy sometimes assumes the sound of a powerful roar of water, while he clearly perceives a sort of great waterfall falling from the Infinite onto the top of his head, inundating him with an ineffable "shining happiness," which has no comparison with any of the pleasures of the senses.

An archetypal reminder of these experiences has evidently remained in the human collective patrimony. In fact, in almost all of the communities with a religious background appears the concept of a river with a sacred character: the Ganges for the Hindus, the Jordan for the Hebrews, the Columbia for the tribes of the American West (Sri Yukteswar's *The Holy Science*).

it touches the upper *Chakra*. When this conjunction has occurred, individual consciousness and consciousness of the species identify the one into the other with an extraordinary expansion of self-awareness (*see* Chapter Two).

In such a man, there is no more feeling of particularistic love with a family, tribe or any other egocentric kind of love, but to him everything is universal in dimensions: he loves all men only because of the fact they are men, that is, creatures of his same species, intended and created by God. We have come to Love with the capital "L," Universal Love, whence the law of Nonviolence (*ahiṃsā*) is directly descended: How can someone be violent, if all are brothers? In its human sense, *ahiṃsā* is therefore but the Hindu equivalent of the Christian Commandment: "Love your neighbor as you love yourself." "Improve yourself," adds Yoga in accordance with Christian mysticism, "and because of this same fact, you will help your fellow man"; "if you do not love yourself enough to want the supreme blessing of spiritual perfection for yourself, how can you sincerely wish for the good of your fellow man?"*

How can man control the tremendous power concealed inside *kuṇḍalinī*? Hindu philosophy thinks that man can reach the control of his genital power in observance of the natural laws, by learning in the course of his life, to channel his sexual energy into activities other than sex. By degrees, and with the exercise of his will, he can (1) transform his sexual energy into physical energy, by training his body to manual work and to the practice of sporting exercises; (2) sublimate the power of sex into power of his mind, for the creation of works of art and science (3) concentrate his sexual energy along with all other forms of vital energy, in order to lift himself up toward Cosmic Consciousness. A trained Yogi knows how to achieve mastery over the sexual drives through voluntary control of the *mūlādhāra* sacral center.

The ancient system of the Hindu society codified in the *Vedas,* vivid traces of which are still existing in modern India, suggests an individual and social training program for man that faithfully reflects its philosophical conception regarding

* "... Therefore be perfect, as your Heavenly Father is perfect" (Matt. 5:48).

the individual and the species. This integral training program
provides for three stages of development, each of which occu-
pies about twenty years of human life. Man should spend the
first twenty years of his life as *brahmachary,* that is, student,
student not in the superficial school meaning, but in the strict
concept of *Haṭha* Yoga, in which, beside formal education, the
training and the purification of the body and mind are taken
care of. Manual work, carried out in the *ashram,* has a great
importance at this stage of training.

The *ashram* is an organization typical of the Hindu educational conception. It lies between the American college and
the hermitage. In an *ashram,* students and Masters live together,
joined by an equal discipline and mutual service. The Master
lavishes the student with his teaching, and the *brahmachary*
tills the soil, whence he gets the nourishment for himself and
for his Master.* As soon as he has acquired sufficient self-
control, the *brahmachary* can get married, and thus comply
with his duty to the species. He then becomes a "Householder"
(Family Father or Mother), keeping the educational spirit,
received in the *ashram,* in the domestic life. This could not be
better expressed in any other way than in the following words
of the Mahatma Gandhi: "For its existence the World depends
on the Act of Generation, and the World is a reflexion of
God's Glory. The Act of Generation must, therefore, be a
controlled volition for an orderly growth of the World."

In the Hindu cosmological conception, a state of purity of
body and of mind in the Father and in the Mother at the
moment of the act of generation, their knowledge of admin-
istering a "rite of universal importance," has a great influence
on the spiritual character of the child who shall be born.

---

* In his attempt to reform India's entire social life, restoring it to its
historical values after the long night of foreign domination, Gandhi pas-
sionately called his fellow countrymen back to the ancient educational tradition. He himself founded an *Ashram*—the famous *Ashram* of Wharda—
where he lavished the best of his oral teachings.

All his life, Gandhi preached the usefulness of work in the fields, instructed his disciples to earn their living with the labor of agriculture,
tried to get the ancient artisan art of hand spinning and weaving, the
khadi, revived throughout the country.

For the Hindus, birth and death are but opposite polarities of a single cosmic phenomenon, governed by the Karmic Law of Cosmic Causation. Just as man's psychological attitude at the moment of his death is decisive for the life of his soul in the hereafter,* so the parents' attitude during the germinative act, even if not determinative, holds a great potential value for good and for bad, on the future life of the incarnate soul. The biological laws of heredity regarding matter grant no medical corroboration of this important Hindu assertion, but it is a proved fact that matings between a man and a woman under negative impulses (anger, jealousy, sex lust,) are negatively reflected on the whole gestation period and even on the modalities of the delivery. The attitude of sweet expectation of a serene spouse who sets about giving birth to a wanted child, is quite different from the attitude of a woman who has been left pregnant by chance, during immoderate sexual activity. Medical statistics have not yet gone, and cannot go, beyond the first days of life of a new-born baby, but I am certain that if the life of children conceived and born under different psychological conditions of the parents could be followed, one could evidence, according to statistical methods, the cosmic truth stated by Hindu philosophy.

The twenty years of life of the *brahmachary* assume, therefore, a deep human meaning for the conscious psychophysical preparation of the future Householder, minister of a rite whose importance is not individual, domestic or tribal, but touches the entire Universe.

When the progeny has been brought up, and his debt toward the species has been discharged, the pious Hindu, before climbing up to the last stage of his earthly education, has the duty to go back to creative study, trying to communicate his lived experience of life to his fellow men, according to his abilities. Only after he has complied with this task can he finally become a *sannhyasin*, that is, a Renouncer of the World. The *sannhyasin* gives up the fruit of his earthly work, and

* ". . . Keep watch therefore, because you don't know when the master of the house will come, whether late at night, at midnight, at the cock-crow, or in the morning; so that, coming suddenly, he won't find you asleep" (Mark 13:35-36).

goes to live with the mate in a retreat, away from the world, leading a frugal life in the mystical practices, in order to complete his spiritual self-realization.

Yoga is the conductor wire and support for man's whole domestic and social education, in Hindu thought. The *brahmachary* draws from Yoga to discipline the body with the *āsanas* and purify the mind with the golden rules of *yama* and *niyama*. The Householder finds in Yoga the ability to subdue sex to an orderly procreation and then reach chastity. In fact, by magnetizing the *mūlādhāra* together with the other *Chakras*, all the sexual energy is concentrated along the cerebro-spinal axis, and is sent to the psyche for total illumination. In this way, the sexual stimulus is subdued and then disappears entirely with absolutely no effort.

Finally, in the practice of *prāṇāyāma*, the *sannhyasin* uses the balmy air, rich in *prāṇa*, of the wood where he lives to reach *pratyāhāra*, the upper stages of *Rāja* Yoga, up to the glorious experience of *samādhi*.

Chapter Seven

Diseases
and Yoga:
A look at our
Disabilities

Pathology means study of diseases, from the Greek words *pathos*—"suffering" and *logos*—"discussion." Clinical pathology is, therefore, an extensive study of diseases as a general phenomenon, which medicine classifies and describes in their characteristics. In the normal man, health is a natural presupposition of the body: when health alters, a disease appears. A disease can assume different characteristics according to the cause, the lesions it causes to the tissues of the organism, the symptoms, the course, and the like. In clinical pathology, therefore, diseases are classified as follows: inflammatory, degenerative, metabolic, endocrine, and so on.

Inflammatory Diseases

The tissues and the organs of the body are extremely jealous of their privacy, so much so that when a foreign body of whatever nature gets into them, at once they react violently in the attempt to kill or expel it. This tissue reaction is called inflammation. The foreign bodies about to cause an inflammatory reaction are many and of different physical and chemical natures. Among them, a particular class is constituted by the microorganisms (bacteria, bacilli, cocci, viruses, and the like), the so-called pathogenous germs, that is, germs able to cause a contagious disease. All the contagious diseases, many of which are certainly well known (e.g., measles, diphtheria, typhus, influenza, pneumonia), fall within the pathology of inflammation.

Inflammation is characterized by a local reaction in the spot where the foreign body has penetrated the tissue, and by a general reaction that the entire organism takes part in, known as fever. Certainly, all of us have experienced a local inflammation because of some superficial skin injury, or because of the prick of a pin, or still other causes. Many of us have also certainly noticed the chief symptoms of the inflammatory reaction: redness, pain, swelling, and trouble in the function of the injured part. A similar local inflammatory reaction takes place inside the body when a microorganism penetrates it, either through the respiratory or digestive systems, or other ways.

Fever is the way in which the entire human organism cooperates with the inflamed part. In its biological meaning, therefore, fever constitutes a reaction beneficial to the recovery of one's health, since it tends to stimulate the whole body to expel the foreign body—or to kill it if it is a pathogenous germ —and to repair the damages caused. Under the stimulus of fever, the metabolism increases, the production of certain hormones increases, in short, the individual energetic patrimony increases to overcome the disease.

After it exceeds a certain variable limit according to the individual resistance, the fever ceases to be a phenomenon useful to the recovery of one's health, and becomes a damage in itself, in that it burns the energetic reserves of the organism, and devitalizes it. . . . Many contagious diseases become deadly not because of the pathogenous germ that has caused them, but because of the reaction it has aroused.

It is known that modern medical therapy limits the damages of the inflammatory reactions to the pathogenous germs by preventing their development within the tissues through the supply of antibiotics, special drugs capable of killing particular microorganisms.

A particular form of inflammation is constituted by the

healing of wounds and by the welding of bone fractures. Here, the organism mobilizes its biological energies through the fever, in order to stimulate the tissues to proliferate and to seal the wound, or to cement one end of a fractured bone to the other. Therefore, it is not the surgeon who heals a wound or a fracture. The surgeon only draws the edges of the wound, or the stumps of the broken bone, close together, then leaves the rest to Mother Nature. A particular form of inflammation is the so-called allergy, that is, a special sensitiveness of the human tissues toward certain substances or atmospheric agents, called allergens: an individual may be allergic to certain substances that cause an inflammatory reaction in his body, but not in the body of other people. A typical allergic reaction is the so-called cold, in which the allergenic agent is the atmospheric cold.

When an inflammatory agent acts for a long period of time on a tissue of the body, and the latter has no great capability of defense, it can lead to chronic inflammation, that is, to an inflammation in which the general reaction of the organism is lacking, there is no fever, but the local symptoms prevail: pain, swelling, functional trouble. Chronic inflammations are to be feared particularly, since they can often be the starting point of the more serious degenerative diseases.

Degenerative Diseases

All of the organs in the body are constituted by particular tissues, different from one another, and united in their task of securing the proper working condition of the organs. To outline an otherwise very complex description, we can picture the organic structure of our body as follows. In every organ, three forms of tissues can be distinguished: an epithelial tissue, which is entrusted with the specific function of the organ (respiratory epithelium of the lung, secretory epithelium of the glands, digestive epithelium of the stomach, and so on), a connective tissue, which is entrusted with a task of support and cementation, a muscular tissue formed by autonomous and striate muscular fibers, which cause the contraction and the relaxation of the organ.

If we compare the human body to a house, we could say that the connective tissue represents the reinforced concrete or brick structure of the building, whereas the epithelium represents the inside of the building, with its heating system, plumbing, sewage, linings and tapestries, furnishings, and the like.

For the good operation of the cells making up the various tissues, and for the harmonious collaboration of the tissues one with the other, the human body must maintain conditions of life, nutrition, elimination, within optimum limits that are very restricted. We have already said that a lack of salt in a man's nutrition is sufficient to kill the organism, the lack of a little iron can cause serious forms of anaemia.

During an entire life span, the organs wear and tear in the course of their function. In part, the wear and tear is made up for by new generations of cells, but beyond a certain limit the equilibrium breaks, the tissues wear out, the organs degenerate. Old age is but a progressive degenerative disease, especially accelerated in man because of his nonnatural habits of life. Observe a 15-year-old cat, how much grace and agility it still has, and then observe a 70-year-old man's behavior, equivalent to the 15-year-old cat on the comparative biological scale. In the former, a more natural life has reduced the degeneration of the tissues; in the latter, an artificial life has enormously quickened the wear and tear of the tissues.

A typical degenerative disease is arteriosclerosis, characterized by a progressive hardening of the walls of the arteries caused by the accumulation in them of cholesterol, a substance derived from the digestion of animal fats. If you stop to think that arteriosclerosis around the world—especially in the countries with a higher standard of life, where people more likely overindulge in the pleasures of the table—*in one year kills more people than past wars did in the same period of time,* you can ponder further on the damages of a faulty nutrition, and on the right Buddhist intuition that has placed the seat of Wisdom in the stomach.

Another frequent degenerative disease is osteoarthritis, which has already been mentioned, due to lack of exercise, nonnatural life, wrong positions of the body, excessive weight, and other factors.

Increasingly, modern medicine points out close connections among psychological attitudes, chronic inflammations, and tissue degeneration. An unharmonious mind, immature and poorly integrated, through the vegetative nervous system, the hormone system, and the somatic system, exerts negative influence on the physical level, causing muscular tension, altered metabolism, diverted hormone production. Consequently, the tissues are deprived of their natural defenses against the attacks of the pathogenous germs, and are subject to small, local, chronic inflammation. These processes keep the cells and tissues of the injured organ in a continuous state of alarm and defense, which hastens their wear and degeneration.

A typical example is the gastric ulcer. Today we know that ulcer of the stomach is a psychosomatic disease, in the sense that its origin can often be traced to a psychological conflict that is projected on the autonomous muscles of the stomach, keeping them in a continuous tension. The muscular tension of the stomach damages the gastric epithelium, which becomes easy prey of the germs brought into the stomach with food, if not damaged by the very gastric juices, which have an acid characteristic. The chronically inflamed epithelium degenerates into a rough scar that contracts the stomach and hampers digestion. Such a poor digestion, from a stomach that does not work at full rhythm, makes the mental condition of an already abnormal patient even worse, in a sequence of causes and effects that can lead to successive tissue degeneration and even death.

Similar psychosomatic processes form the basis for many so-called female sexual troubles, characterized by chronic back aches, aches in the legs, restlessness, insomnia, chronic inflammations of the uterus, and menstrual irregularities.

A particular form of degeneration is constituted by the tumors. In the normal tissues, the cells reproduce methodically, according to the biological needs of the organs, to substitute for other cells, which are dead, or to strengthen the function of a particularly worn organ. In tumors, at a certain point, the cells of a determinate organ become disobedient to the biological laws, and start to proliferate in a disorderly way, with no further consideration for the function of the organ. If this proliferation is limited to a single organ, and still partly respects its function, the tumor will be considered "benign." On the other hand, when the disobedience of the cells respects neither the limits of the human organs nor their function, but spreads everywhere in the body like weeds in the fields, then the tumor is said to be "malignant."

Medicine has not yet discovered the ultimate cause of cellular disobedience, which lies at the basis of a tumor, but has pointed out constant relationships between tissue proliferation and chronic inflammation. In other words, it can happen that cells that are exposed for a long period of time to a chronic inflammatory stimulus "revolt" and start an "anarchic revolution," proliferating like weeds. The dreaded cancer of the stomach, the feared cancer of the tongue, the sly cancer of the lung at their origin often have an inflammatory cause, because of gastric ulcer, sores and trauma in the tongue, inflammation from smoke in the lungs. Statistical data have not proved it, but a cause-effect connection may be likely between forms of tumor and psychological disorders, possibly through areas of chronic inflammation, like ulcer of the stomach.

Metabolic Diseases

In medicine, those diseases that are caused by a disorder of the material metabolism are known as metabolic diseases. In Chapter Three, I tried to give an idea of metabolism in its anabolic and catabolic functions toward the different groups of chemical substances making up the foods we eat. I have compared the chemical structures of the substances to small cube buildings. We can thus say that if something goes wrong in the composition or in the resolution of the small cubes, the disease appears. A well known metabolic disease is diabetes, in which there is a deviation of the sugar metabolism so that the liver can no longer use the sugar conveyed in the blood. The sugar, consequently, accumulates in the blood and in the tissues and chronically intoxicates the organism.

I have already mentioned another typical metabolic disease, gout, due to an accumulation in the kidneys and in the articulations of uric acid, a substance denatured from the catabolism of animal proteins.

But perhaps the most common metabolic disease, even though not always acknowledged as such, is obesity, that is, the excessive accumulation of fat in the body. Many factors can predispose to obesity, especially deficiency of hormone glandular functions, but its prime cause is an alimentary mistake, both quantitative and qualitative: too much food in relation to the kind of life a man leads, especially if he has sedentary and unnatural habits, with too much indulgence toward fats, starches, seasonings, sweets. Obesity represents a serious liability for the general economy of the organism. It imposes overwork on the heart, stuffs the arteries with cholesterol, exposes the articulations to an excessive weight, the liver and the kidneys to a metabolic tear. Statistical data on mortality gathered by insurance companies throughout the world, show that the probability of survival after the middle age *diminishes by 10 percent for every 20 lbs. of body weight in excess* of the optimum average for every individual, in relation to his height and constitution.

Excessive food intake is often sustained by a neurotic appetite, which loses any connection with the metabolic necessities of the organism, and is constantly reinforced by the gratification of the smell and taste senses. Today, obesity is basically viewed as another psychosomatic disorder, where inner mental tensions, arising from a maladjusted personality, are converted into a neurotic appetite, and find expression in overindulgence to the pleasures of the table.

Endocrine Diseases

In Chapter One, I mentioned the endocrine glands and refered to the hormones as quanta of energy, condensed by the glands themselves. The entire organism is placed under the control of the hormones: every system, every organ, every tissue, even every cell is guided in its function by a hormone in collaboration with the vitamins (other quanta of biological energy) and the oligo-minerals.

The endocrine diseases are the consequence either of the deficiency of one or more glands, or of a functional excess of the same. In the first case, we have a reduction of the functions controlled by the gland, in the second case, a functional excitement will result.

The thyroid, for example, regulates organic metabolism. Consequently, its hormone deficiency is characterized by a drop of the metabolic values, a slackening of the vital functions, and the fragility of the entire organism, as happens in the so-called hypothyroid cretinism. On the contrary, an excessive production of the thyroid hormone (Basedow's disease) excites metabolism, with an accelerated activity of the heart, of the muscles, of the nervous system. The Basedowian is an individual in continuous psychomotory agitation, dangerously emotional, reacting confusedly, like a utility passenger car burning the kerosene of a jet engine, as fuel. The waste of energy is tremendous and useless, ultimately burning out the life of the patient.

I have tried to give an idea of the most common diseases affecting man, their causes and their modalities. I will now attempt a more comprehensive synthesis, useful for what we still have to say on this subject.

Health is a divine privilege granted by the Creator to all living creatures, provided they respect the Laws of Nature. Look at the animals, especially the not too tame ones (that is, humanized): Have you ever seen them obese, arteriosclerotic, gouty? Observe how rapidly and with little inflammation cats recover even from their most serious wounds, without disinfectants, antibiotics, or surgeons who sew their wounds up. Why? Because the wild animal, by instinct, obeys the Laws of Nature; man does not.

Diseases, all diseases, are the product of certain constant factors: an artificial environment, an unhealthy conduct of life, a disharmonious mental equilibrium. Because of these common denominators, all the diseases described by pathology present common characteristics. An unhealthy artificial environment multiplies the number of the pathogenous germs and of other accidental inflammatory causes. The inflammation assembles the biological energies of the organism to eliminate the very cause of the inflammation. But if the vital energies, in turn, are reduced because of an unnatural life, the inflammation becomes chronic and leads to the degeneration of the tissues and of the organs. The degeneration of an organ signifies the biological impoverishment of the individual who will thus be even weaker and readier to fall ill. The endocrine glands try to compensate for the lack of balance by supplying extra energetic labor, until even they wear out and add their deficit to the general deficiency of the organism. One more small inflammation, and it will be the end.

You might think this view pessimistic or that I exaggerate.

Shall we consider a few examples drawn from common every-day experience?

A boy wishes to play the "be-a-man game" before his time has come, and smokes a few cigarettes. His bronchi are irritated by the smoke, and at the first germ infiltrating them with the smoky air of the city a nasty bronchitis occurs. It heals, but a small center of chronic inflammation remains. The bronchial and the nearby pulmonary epithelium degenerate into a circumscribed region, and do not seem to give any trouble, but the first Kock's bacillus happening by will find an ideal ground to multiply in, and the first tuberculous center appears. If the individual does not realize it in time, and does not radically change his way of life, the center expands, the bacilli go into the blood, stop in the bones, in the kidneys, in the intestines, and proliferate: organs, tissues, and entire organic systems degenerate, the glands wear out, and death follows prematurely. Following chronic inflammation of the bronchi from smoke, one day the cells of these air pipes may decide to go on strike and start a big protest, otherwise known as cancer of the lung; or the muscles of the bronchi may degenerate to the point where the poor fellow chokes to death in what medicine calls obstructive pulmonary disease (emphysema), in a slow process of breathing impairment that is almost the opposite of *Prāṇāyāma*.

A man full of health, a true "jolly good fellow," enjoys life and its pleasures, having a predilection for the pleasures of the table. His weight increases, but his health is excellent and his work is going fine. Then one nasty day, the epithelium of his stomach, too tired from digesting piles of food, falls prey to a small inflammation. A small gastritis, a few days of alimentary penance, a few pills, and all is over. But in the privacy of the epithelium, the chronic inflammatory center remains. The next germ arriving with a good custard-pie will no longer be the cause of a slight gastritis, but of a violent Staphylococcus gastroenteritis with high fever and energetic mobilization of the entire organism. But the heart, tired of pumping blood into a body which is too fat, the liver, tired of taking on fat with the food swallowed in too large quantities, no longer respond to the energetic requests, wear out and degenerate; consequence: invalidity or death.

On the other hand, another man overindulges in the pleasures of sex, but keeps within the limits of a fairly healthy diet. However, the excessive energy consumption required by the sexual abuse demands a greater contribution of energy. Our man resorts to alcohol. At first, only a few small glasses, then more and more, as an essential side-dish to the pleasures of the senses. His stomach suffers because of too much alcohol, causing a small chronic inflammation, a heartburn after meals, which disappears with a few small drops of wine. The step from small inflammation to alcoholic degeneration of the liver is long but certain. Meanwhile, alcohol alters the cognitive faculties of the mind, so that our man deludes himself with more alcohol: His liver swells, his heart suffers, his mind becomes dull. Nobody knows which shall kill the poor man first: Will it be the alcoholized heart and liver, the auto accident, or just any other factor arising from chronic alcoholism?

Health professionals fight a losing battle against disease. Even though they might eliminate a certain pathological symptom, they do not and cannot heal, just as social psychology cannot teach morality. Both are transitory activities, extrinsic to man. In the medical cure a close adherence of a man to his health is missing; man lacks the will power to live a natural life, the only true bulwark against diseases. Men would like to enjoy their health without earning it, just as they wish for Paradise in the Hereafter, without moral commitment in this life.

Drugs are toxic substances, which, within recommended doses, perform certain useful actions: They relax tense muscles, dilate or contract the arteries, depress or stimulate the function of the heart, stomach, or other organs. They soothe or stimulate the nervous system; they kill a few billion microorganisms, and so on. But they do this through an external, artificial mechanism whose effect is transitory, and potential damage from accumulation is always possible. The drug does not require the adherence of the individual to his recovery, but simply eliminates temporarily the symptoms of a disease. If recovery follows the suppression of the symptoms, it is not the drug that has worked it, just as it was not the surgeon who healed the wound. The real healer was Nature, which for a moment was able to recover sufficient energy, taking advantage of the forced rest imposed on the patient either because of a sedative, pain, or other reason. The real recovery from any disease consists in the healing of the human disharmonies. To join man's separate parts together again, to subject the function of the body to the control of the mind, in an intelligent expression of emotions, to put at the disposal of the entire human entity a biological energy patrimony no longer scattered in a thousand mistakes of life, but concentrated to fight and to eliminate eventual and residual causes of disease consciously—this is the real recovery of man.

The Hindu point of view in problems of health and disease has been elaborated throughout the centuries, along the Vedic tradition of intuitive knowledge and wisdom, tested on practical experience. The medicophilosophical concepts contained in the *Vedas* have been translated in modern Yoga teaching, with a terminology to suit the intellect of present-day men.

In Chapter One, I mentioned the *Chakras,* placed along the cerebrospinal axis as six centers of concentration and of irradiation of the "pranic" energy reaching man through breathing, food, sun radiations. Since every *Chakra* has a double polarity, one positive and one negative, all the *Chakras* together form sort of a great electrical wire along the vertebral column, covered by a current of energy with a positive sign, which goes down from the upper *Chakra* to the lower one, and a current bearing the negative sign, which climbs upward. The positive current, according to Yoga, "gives life," whereas the negative current "receives and sustains the vital phenomena."*

Modern physiology has experimentally confirmed this ancient intuition of the Hindus, showing that all the vital phenomena of the organism are characterized by variations of electric potentials, from positive to negative, and vice versa. The nervous fibers, the vegetative ganglia, the muscles, the cells of every tissue, are electrically neutral when they are in a state of rest. They charge positively during the first stage of activity,

---

* The universally known emblem of the medical science is a twig round which are twined two small snakes. It symbolizes this Hindu conception, for the twig represents the "tree of life," that is, the vertebral column, and the two small snakes are the two currents of pranic energy, *pingala* and *iḍa,* flowing up and down along the spinal cord.

negatively during the second stage, and again become electrically neutral in the following short period of rest. The positive-
negative electric phases are essential to a correct operation of
all the organs. Any alteration leads to a functional lack of
balance. For example, many muscle-relaxants eliminate the
muscular tone by interfering with the electric potentials at the
level of the neuromotor plate. On the contrary, by stimulating
a muscle with electric current too long, the muscle becomes
tetanic, that is, it gets into spastic contraction and cannot function any longer.

The sages of ancient India not only intuitively sensed that
life is basically an electrical phenomenon, but from it they
drew the practical conclusion that health is the result of a
harmonious balance between positive and negative electric
forces, properly distributed along the three dimensions of the
human body: the somatic, the vegetative, and the hormone
systems.

The supreme regulator for the distribution of vital energy
in man is the Mind-power. The better it is adjusted, the better
it can distribute the energy, regulating the needs of the three
parts. On the other hand, a consciousness "in the dark," identified in only one part of the body, carries out its tasks of life
and health in a disorderly way. An open Mind generally
induces a slight prevalence of positive energy, through positive
thinking. Positive energy vitalizes the body. In physiological
terms, this means vegetative and hormone activities smartly
adjusted to meet all the individual needs on the somatic level.
An excessive expansion of Mind-power in relation to the state
of vitality of the body, that is, a too intensive electropositive
prevalence, can lead to a frailness of health and to a certain
weakness of the body. This is a phenomenon well known to
the Disciples-Yogis and to the mystics of every religion taking
their first steps. As their consciousness expands, and their living refines, surprisingly they feel various troubles in their
body that did not exist before. Organs and systems get delicate
in their operations—a stomach already able to digest any food
now revolts if subjected to alimentary immoderation. Some of
the diseases recorded in the lives of saints were probably due
to an excessive spiritual force not matched by adequate physical training.

It happens as though the Consciousness, "overlighted" in relation to the body, were sending to the nervous network a current tension that the system is not prepared to uphold: Here and there some fuses can "blow." For this reason, the spiritual ascent of *Rāja* Yoga is always coupled with a severe physical training according to the precepts of *Haṭha* Yoga, so that the conscious mental development is harmoniously matched by an equally conscious physical development: "Conscious health, conscious vitality, conscious fulfillment" are the three prayers of the *Rāja* Yogi.

On the contrary, a limited Mind-power with large dark areas produces negative energy. Negative energy devitalizes the body. Physiologically, this means a reduction of the neurovegetative and hormone activities. The organism operates within limits below its possibilities. Man's entire attitude regarding life becomes negative. A further reduction of Consciousness will undoubtedly lead to abnormality and diseases.

There are men and women whose vital energy seems to disperse mysteriously. They are always weary people who at the least strain, at the slightest hitch, lose heart, at the first pain give up. They are prey to infections, which in them always assume serious and complicated courses. Physicians and surgeons alike are wary of these persons, knowing by experience their frailness and their lack of resistance. A disease that in others responds quickly, in these wretched people gives rise to all sorts of complications. A surgical operation, ordinarily quite safe, develops in one of these negatives in a strangely stormy manner: the surgical wound will not heal and festers, the intestines will not stir, the kidneys do not work properly, blood pressure subsides, the body loses strength, and the mind grows dim. Sometimes death follows.

To the same class of negative people belongs another group of persons in whom the exact opposite seems to happen, where the vital energy assumes a destructive power, like the power latent in a volcano. These are the everlasting unlucky people, the chronic "busters." If they stir, they break something; if they drive, they cause damages to themselves or to others, even though they want to be careful; if they work, they overdo it, and do it wrong; even when they are on a vacation, they absolutely must bustle about, be always on the go. Despite their apparent exuberant vitality, these people are not more resistant than the negatives to disease and pain. When they are taken ill, they react as they have always reacted in life, violently: great fevers, scars disproportionate to the wound, huge bony spurs following small fractures, inflammations. When the reactive violence used during the first days of a disease fails to restore health, these people lose heart and become perhaps weaker and more dangerous than other negative people: they literally expire like a lamp whose fuel has run out.

The secret for the cure of these wretched negative people lies not in the body nor in the unconscious, but in Consciousness. Psychoanalysis cannot cure them with its approaches. Only a personal, volitional, and conscious effort, following the precepts of Yoga or of any other serious school of spiritual Mystical training, is able to start that almost miraculous ascending spiral through which Mind-power vitalizes the body and the energized body supplies extra energy to the Mind for the subsequent stages of Self-Realization. On the spiritual path, healing is therefore achieved naturally, as a consequence of the reunion of the mind with the body.

In keeping with their doctrine of biological bipolarity, Vedic India's ancient sages classified man's diseases "positive" or "negative," according to the prevalence of positive or negative energy in the body. Let us resume this classification within the frame of clinical pathology.

Positive Diseases

Positive diseases can include all the diseases from inflammation, where there is a reaction of positive defense of the organism to eliminate the inflammatory agent and overcome the disease. But fever, the greatest reactive expression of the body, in itself can be a waste of energy. The well-known shiver accompanying the fever is but an unconscious subliminal muscular contraction, changing the polarity to negative. This change causes chronic inflammation and degeneration of the tissues, devitalizing the cells.

Western physicians cure the diseases from inflammation by two methods: fever-fighting drugs and antibiotics. The evolved Yogi attains the same result in two ways of conscious self-control. He reduces any waste of energy through a complete muscular relaxation, then hypervitalizes the part of his body struck by the inflammation, by mentally concentrating on it the vital energy stored in the *Chakras*. The tissues thus energized can biologically destroy the inflammatory agent, or eject it more actively. In a sense, this hypervitalization mentioned by Yoga would be but an increase of the immunity powers of the human body. Among the positive diseases can be included certain forms of excessive cellular activity in some tissues and organs (allergies? Collagen diseases?), some disfunctions of the rhythm of the heart, of the circulation, of the nervous system. Instead of taking sedative drugs or tranquillizers, the Yogi consciously inhibits himself through *Pratyahara,* and diminishes the activity of the entire organism.

Negative Diseases

Obviously, diseases with a negative polarity are all the forms of degeneration of the tissues, some metabolic diseases, as well as many hormone diseases, characterized by a defect of function or by an immoderate hyperactivity (Cushing's disease, acromegaly, gigantism). A disharmonious Mind-power may explain both the prevalence of the negative energy in the body and the poor ability of the patient to attain recovery consciously. In the mature Yogi, a negative disease is less likely, since in him *yama* and *niyama* have already worked the necessary purifications of the body and of the mind. In any case, once the control of the vital energy is acquired, it is possible to magnetize the *Chakra,* on which the function of the sick organ depends, and send a wave of vitalizing positive energy to it.

To many readers, this will seem somewhat theoretical, and maybe they will think that the business of magnetizing the *Chakras* to cure illnesses is something similar to Icarus' Utopia. I don't deny the difficulty of mastery of one's body. It is also a historical fact that fully evolved Yogis have died of diseases, even though here perhaps there are metaphysical factors it is not our task to discuss. I wish, however, to invite my readers to a small reflection. Have you ever noticed how very seldom a person is taken ill on the eve of a very important event of his life? Have you ever observed how a cold, an influenza with a slight persistent fever, a small back ache, disappear

almost by magic the day of one's wedding, or the day one has
to leave for a long-wished vacation, or for other similar happy
reasons in our daily lives? What happened? Unconsciously, the
Chakras have been magnetized. The Mind, strained to its
maximum to attain the longed-for goal, has discharged a strong
current of positive energy into the vegetative plexuses, for a
moment the cells and the tissues have been vitalized and have
been able to eliminate the disease. Perhaps one thanks the
drugs one has taken on the eve of one's vacation for the gained
recovery. One forgets that no drug can heal; only Nature,
that is, our real "I," our full Will Power, can draw from
Nature the vital energy able to heal. The physicians of ancient
India were not the only ones to say it. Any physician of any
country in the world has had this experience, and has learned
to fear it or to use it to a good purpose, according to his
patient's state of mind.

The rules contained in *yama* and *niyama*, as well as the
practice of the *āsanas*, constitute per se a precious health
insurance, apart from their value as steps of the spiritual training. They teach alimentary and sexual continence, they train
the disciple to be self-controlled, balanced and generous in
every life situation; they emphasize outdoor life, with frequent
exposures to the rays of the sun; they prescribe a whole series
of simple psychophysical techniques, designed to meet all the
health requirements of our body. If only for this immense
benefit offered to all men, Yoga deserves to be known better
and appreciated more. It is not the selfish quest for occult
powers that should propel people on the Yogic path, but first
the most elementary and natural aspiration: the health of the
mind and of the body, as it was bestowed on us by our Creator.
Yoga teaches that the human body is the vehicle through
which we express ourselves as souls. The preservation of health
is consequently our first duty, if we want to achieve any spiritual goal. By the same token, body discipline, which is the
first prerequisite for health, cannot be enforced without striv-
ing to grow better in our inner spiritual nature.

Modern physical therapy has developed many techniques of
mental and physical rehabilitation, which have much in common with Yogic principles of health training. However,
between physiotherapy and Yoga there is the same difference

as there is between calisthenic exercises and the *āsanas*: The former are transitory processes requiring only the adherence of the body; Yoga directly requires the complete and active adherence of the body and of the mind, in harmonious coordination with each other. Only recently, contemporary physical therapy has become aware of the key rôle of educating the mind of the patient into positive thinking, in order to achieve long-lasting results in rehabilitation programs. In almost all the Departments of Physical Therapy in the United States, teams of psychologists do work with the physiotherapists to achieve a balanced psychosomatic recovery of the diseased patient.

To conclude, let us try to imagine the advantages that the "jolly good fellow," the fat and gluttonous man of the example given in the preceding pages, can obtain from Yoga.

If one day this man, alarmed by his excessive body weight, or worried by small ailments which, after the last plateful of lobster, still remain in spite of the many pills he has gulped down, or even bothered by some small trouble of a not well-defined moral conscience; if one day this man made a firm decision to change his life, and chose *Haṭha* Yoga as his school of self-reform, this is approximately what would happen.

Most probably, our man would start his work by trying to perform some simple *āsana* copied from one of the many popular books on Yoga. During the first days, he would gain nothing but a few pains in the articulations, a few tumbles from the less easy positions, and a subjective feeling of being all broken. Able to persevere, after a few weeks, he would notice something new and nimble in his entire behavior. His articulations will have become soft as they haven't been for years, his backbone straightened up and become more flexible in its movements, his face more relaxed. Slowly, he will perform his *āsanas*, better and better, and venture into something more difficult.

Made trustful of Yoga, our man would begin to probe the subject, and from the simple popularized booklet, he would climb to more binding philosophical and literary sources, discover and eventually practice the rules of *yama* and *niyama*.

At first, he will start to eliminate from his table the heavier foods: pork, meat-pies, and the like. After the first 10 pounds of weight he loses, he will feel like a new man, with a greater vitality, a clearer mind, a more youthful behavior. To his surprise, he will notice that the less he eats, the less he wants to eat. No longer the slave of his stomach, he will turn into the master of his former tyrant, and satisfy his hunger as required by his metabolic necessities. Subsequently, he eliminates from his diet every kind of meat, the excesses of noodles, fats, and sweets, giving his preference to vegetables, fruits, and cereals. Another 20 pounds of body weight thus vanish, with no effort. One more little step, and the habit of the alcoholic beverages disappears: only a glass of light wine with meals is more than sufficient! Our good friend now looks like the son of himself.

Meanwhile, he is undergoing a year of regular training: fifteen minutes every morning and every evening, he has almost reached the mastery of all the *āsanas.* Now his articulations bend submissive in the *padnāsana* position, allowing him a few minutes of complete psychophysical relaxation. Then one day, to his pleasant surprise, he will discover he can without effort perform the most glamorous of the *āsanas,* the *śirśāsana,* and remain upside-down a few minutes without miserably crashing to the floor, as it used to happen.

But the fact that he knows how to perform *padnāsana* and *śirśāsana* would mean nothing if it were not coupled by another important discovery. Our man, the ex-"jolly good fellow," is beginning to experience a new joy, much more beautiful and more lasting than the one he used to relish through his palate. He is enjoying peace of mind. Acquiring the control of his stomach, overcoming his predominant bad habit, gluttony, it seems that all the other bad habits have gone by magic. He finds it easier to control anger, jealousy, and other passions torturing him before. Freed from the poisons of gluttony, relieved from those of envy and sloth, his body enters a harmonious state never enjoyed before; his heart pumps blood freely and quietly into arteries that have become elastic and cleared of impurities; his liver works at a minimum of wear; his kidneys are at rest; his lungs submit to the practice of *prāṇāyāma;* all the economy of the organism has been reorganized and revitalized. Consequently, the mind is clearer, readier, more open. Consciousness starts to shine and a positive energy prevails where before it was all negative. Now disease, no matter how serious, will find cells, tissues, and organs full of vitality and ready to overcome the invasion in a short time, where before it could have been a matter of life or death.

And so, the ex-glutton is dead. In his place is born the new Man, moving toward the attainment of higher spiritual goals. If in his heart there is the sincere desire to evolve further, he will find a spiritual teacher—a *guru* as they call him in India —who will lead him by the hand to the only, truly real goal granted to man: Realization in Cosmic Consciousness.

Health Science is growing aware that injuries and diseases are not mere accidents of our material life, but that they are someway influenced by subtle electromagnetic forces, of which we are totally unconscious. "Invisible rhythms underlie most of what we assume to be constant in ourselves and the world around us. . . . Though we can neither see nor feel them, we are surrounded by forces of gravity, electromagnetic fields, light waves, air pressure, sound waves. . . . Undulatory cycles are the most usual, yet overlooked, property of earth life. . . ." These words are not from the *Upanishads,* but they are quoted from a 1970 publication of the U.S. National Institute of Mental health.*

Psychology to-day speaks of "Circadian Rhythms" (from the latin words: *circam dies,* around-day) to indicate those undulatory changes in body activities that seem to be influenced by daily variations in atmospheric pressure, light and darkness, electromagnetic forces. It also speaks of "Infradian Rhythms" in reference to cycles longer than circadian, such as weeks and months.

A large amount of research has shown that many biological functions, such as enzyme production, hormone outputs, metabolic activities, blood cell production, are exhibiting the same rhythmic undulations of our planet as it turns on its axis and around the sun.

Circadian and Infradian Rhythms in our biological functioning mean that there are periods of maximum strength or weakness in our mental and physical performances, which

* "Biological Rhythms in Psychiatry and Medicine," U.S. Department of Health, Education, and Welfare, Public Health Service Publication No. 2088.)

subtlely influence our responses to every kind of stress in our daily living. For each day, week, and month, there are hours when we are stronger, have a greater understanding and endurance, even hours of higher immunity. There are also rhythms in the toxicity of pharmaceutical drugs, which means that timing often makes the difference between beneficial or harmful effects of any given common drug. A number of well-known physical and mental diseases, such as menstrual syndromes, hypertension, gastric ulcers, manic depression, have been already shown to be influenced by undulatory cycles, obviously in connection with changes in biological functions.

In my own opinion, the most fascinating of contemporary scientific investigations seems to be the study of the pineal gland in relation to the possible role it plays in biological rhythmicity. The pineal gland is a little, pine-coned structure with several sympathetic nervous fibers, situated deeply in the middle of the brain, between the two cerebral hemisphere. This gland is often referred in modern Yogic teaching as the physical counterpart of the so-called "spiritual eye" or "third eye," whose projection is felt in deep meditation on the forehead, between the eyebrows. References to the "Spiritual eye" are found both in the *Bhagavad Gita* and in the Bible.*

So far the biological function of this gland is poorly understood. By present-day evidence, Western thought refers to the pineal gland as a kind of biological clock, possibly influenced by changes of light and darkness through the optic nerve tracts and the sympathetic system. With the discovery of biological rhythmicity, Western science has crossed the ages and reached to the Vedic concept of "duality" in the relative worlds of creation, expressed in the laws of *māyā* and *karma*.†

---

* ("The light of the body is the eye. If therefore thine eye be single, thy whole body shall be full of light." Matthew 6/22)

† *See: Autobiography of a Yogi*, by Paramahansa Yogananda. (26)

Chapter Eight

What Pain is:
A look
at Human
Suffering

More than two thousand years ago, Aristotle called men's pain "a wailing of the soul." In more recent times, the great neurophysiologist Dr. Sherrington defined pain as a "mental elaboration of an imperative protective reflex."

Both definitions, and many other more or less dramatic statements from philosophers and scientists in the course of the centuries, want to point out the essential fact that human pain is not a simple physiological sensation, like a sixth sense in man, but a complex phenomenon in which the whole human psychosomatic nature is revealed.

In the course of our lives, we all have experienced some pains and aches, and consequently we think we all know the unpleasant aspects of pain, but if we go a little deeper into the phenomenon of pain, we should probably realize how little we actually know about this experience so important in our lives.

Let me offer a little example to illustrate this point better. If you burn your hand while holding a hot paper cup of coffee in a campground, you are likely to simply drop it and shake your hand. But if you feel the same burning from your hot paper cup while standing on a very precious oriental rug in the home of your boss, or while handling an expensive piece of china, you are not likely to simply drop the offending cup, but rather you first *will put it down safely and then you will shake your hand*. In other words, you have quickly evaluated your unpleasant feeling not only in terms of damage to your hand, but also in connection with environmental and affective factors.

What is pain then? Is it a simple perception based on sensory data, or is it a complex emotional and behavioral phenomenon? Let us examine it briefly, in order to extract from this analysis some elements for further discussion according to this book's thesis.

A Neurological Outline

Contemporary neurophysiologists think that the sensory impulses generating the painful perception (*see* Chapters One and Two) are transmitted along two different lines of nerve fibers. One line is a fast transmitter so that impulses traveling along it "ring the bell" quickly, alerting the brain that something is hurting us. The second line is a slow transmitter. Its signals are not designed to give information about the "hurt," but to trigger an emotional reaction to it. You can demonstrate this dual transmission the next time you hammer your thumb. If you keep cool and watch yourself, you will notice first a sharp, lightening perception of the hurt. Then, a few moments later, a throbbing, highly unpleasant ache will prompt you to moan, groan, call for help, for attention, for "tender loving care," and so on. In other words, upon perceiving the "second pain," you will manifest it emotionally.

A decade ago, two scientists, Melzack and Wall, proposed an interesting theory about pain in connection with its dual transmission. It is worth mentioning here, since it comes close to the Yoga points of view. It is called the "Spinal-Gate Theory," and could be presented as follows: In the spinal cord we have some neurological mechanisms that could be spoken of as a gate control. When the gate is open, all the painful impulses can go through and reach the brain; when it is closed, few or no impulses are allowed through. There are two "keys for the spinal gate": one key is held by the set of fast-transmitting nerve fibers that "ring the bell" in the brain; the second key is held by those nerve fibers that come down from the brain centers to the spinal gate, carrying to it impulses elaborated upon by emotional processes. These emotional drives have been triggered by the first "ringing" of the painful bell, that is, the hurt, but are further sustained by the secondary unpleasant impulses reaching the brain over the slow-transmitting network.

In the above example of the hot cup of coffee, the fact that you didn't drop it on the expensive rug could be explained according to the "Gate Theory," as follows: Upon perceiving the burning hurt, you quickly evaluated the possible consequences of spilling the coffee over your boss' rug, and consequently your emotional brain centers "closed the gate," shutting further painful impulses out, until the cup was safely put down.

The "Spinal-Gate Theory" seems to explain in refined neurological terms the well-known fact that many people under strong emotional drives have shown little or no experience of pain—prisoners tortured by a cruel enemy, who were able to stand a great deal of suffering without giving up, ancient and modern religious martyrs who went to painful death almost in a triumphant way, soldiers wounded on the battlefield, who were able to walk out of the danger areas despite serious body lesions, and so on. All these people were able to overcome momentarily the painful experience, probably closing their "spinal gate" to all sensory inputs. Diagram D. tries to present a visual outline of the "Spinal-Gate" mechanism.

The "Spinal-Gate Theory" proposed by Melzack and Wall also offers an explanation of possible differences between animals' and men's pain responses. The animal accepts the pain as a physical sensation, but does not elaborate upon it, and probably has a primitive spinal-gate control. A dog perceiving a hurt while in a room full of good food (for him), will not hesitate to waste it all, in order to quickly escape the hurt. We don't. We will always elaborate our hurts emotionally, and are likely to put in the experience our entire personality.

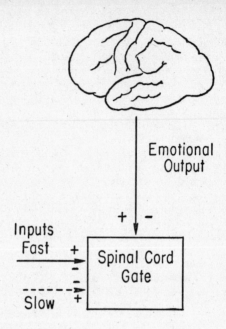

The spinal gate theory

DIAGRAM D The "Spinal Gate" is opened and closed by two different control sets: (1) the fast sensory inputs to the spinal cord; (2)
the nerve impulses from the brain centers to the neurological mechanisms of the "gate." When the "gate" is too open, all the slow
sensory inputs are allowed through and go to the brain, where they
are perceived as highly unpleasant sensations. In turn, such "nox-
ious" perceptions deeply disturb the balance of our brain functions,
and are likely to trigger sets of impulses from the brain to the "spinal
gate," further upsetting its delicate control mechanisms.

The "Spinal Gate Theory" is, so far, the best neurological explanation of the Yogic capability to isolate the perceptive brain centers
from the outer sensory stimulations. We can represent this capability
as inhibition of the "spinal gate," achieved via strong volitional
impulses from the brain to the "gate" mechanisms in the spinal cord.

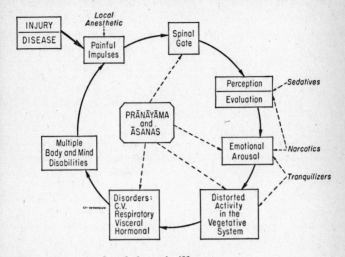

The vicious cycle of chronic illness

DIAGRAM E Painful impulses, on reaching the brain after having been modulated through the "spinal gate," are perceived and evaluated, and trigger an emotional arousal. If not properly checked through an orderly rational and volitional control, the emotional reaction may induce and sustain abnormal activities within the vegetative system, mostly sympathetic (*see also* Chapters One and Seven). As a consequence, various disorders in the heart, arteries and veins, hormones, and other various viscera are produced; each one in turn induces further mental and physical disabilities. A vicious circle of pain and sickness is generated in this way, with more painful impulses further deteriorating the emotional stability of the sufferer.

Sedative drugs probably act in reducing the perceptive evaluation of the painful impulses. Narcotics and tranquillizers slow down and dull both the emotional arousal and the consequent sympathetic distorted activities. All these drugs, however, act in negative ways, practically poisoning the nervous structures into inactivity. *Āsanas* and *prāṇāyāma*, on the other hand, act upon the same nervous stations in positive ways, bringing the emotional responses to pain under the control of cognition and volition, and rehabilitating the neurovegetative system to function properly again. Moreover, *prāṇāyāma* can gain control of the "gate," consequently breaking through whatever vicious circle of chronic illness that might have been generated.

It has been said that man pays with greater suffering for
his more flawless central nervous structure. I think that man
pays with more pain because he refuses to use properly his
refined nervous system, keeping it unbalanced and out of
control.

Each individual interprets pain in relation to his own
cognitive and emotional faculties, in connection with memories of past experiences, environmental factors, and/or in the
fear of further unpleasant perceptions.

Generically speaking, the more the personality is harmonious, the better it can respond to pain as to any other stimulus
inside or outside. On the contrary, a "dark" mind will tend
to interpret pain on the basis of its own conflicts. Thus, for
example, an extroverted man becomes upset under the stimulus of pain, wails, cries out in a loud voice for help from
the outside, whereas an introverted individual will rather
withdraw to himself under the pressure of pain, be subject
to inner worries, perhaps considering pain a punishment for
assumed guilts, secretly enjoying it, almost to the limits of
an unconscious sadism.

In medicine, there are certain pathological processes, called
"vicious circles," in which a functional disturbance causes a
second one, the second one leads to a third one, and so forth,
until the first disturbance becomes worse and is made irrevers-
ible. Something similar happens in the pain syndromes: A
painful perception, when it is intense and lasts enough time,
becomes a source of chronic irritation and, as a consequence,
causes spasms of the arteries and of the muscles, visceral disorders, alterations in the hormone production, increasing
emotional unbalance, with a fatal aggravation of the primitive pain syndrome.

In other words, in intense or chronic pain syndromes, the
vegetative and the hormonal systems join the somatic system
in their various responses to the emotional elaboration of the
painful perception. In consequence, the blood pressure may
increase; nausea, vomiting, and other stomach upsets can
appear; the liver may "go on strike" with a metabolic deficiency; the production of many hormones may be increased
or impaired.

In Chapter Five, I pointed out that breathing constitutes

the most immediate natural link connecting the different parts of the human psychophysical whole. We can now understand how pain, on a different level of physiology, can become another not less direct and powerful link joining man's rent parts. In fact, when pain appears, the three physical systems of the individual are summoned to solidarity with each other and with the mind, to meet the challenge presented by the injury or the disease.

Let us quickly outline how this happens, according to modern medical concepts.

A Clinical Outline of Pain

For the sake of a simple description, here I shall mention three principal forms of common pain syndromes, seen with the eye of a physician.

1. *Surface Pain.* It includes the painful syndromes caused by agents at the level of the skin or of the mucous membranes. The painful stimulus can be physical (burns, frost-bites), chemical (chemical scalds), mechanical (stings, wounds, lacerations, etc.). In every case, there is pain with unmistakable characteristics: sharp, stinging, stimulating a prompt reaction of defense that can be located in every spot of the body. Each one of us has certainly experienced this kind of pain.

2. *Deep Pain.* It is characterized by a dull, diffuse sensation, one that is barely located, almost always coupled by muscular spasm. Unlike the surface pain, which stimulates to a quick reaction, deep pain involves a series of depressing phenomena (nausea, perspiration, fainting fits, etc.) to which could be attached a protective meaning in that they compel the patient to rest and stay quiet. Deep pain is caused by chemical or physical stimuli of the bones, articulations, muscles, nerves, which give rise to somatic pain syndromes, or by the straining, twisting, or contraction of some internal organs, causing visceral pain syndromes (which involve the heart, the liver, the stomach, etc.).

3. *Referred Pain.* This term is used to indicate a pain far removed from the place of primitive pain stimulation. It is but a form of deep somatic and visceral pain, perceived not so much in the point of the stimulus as in an area of projection far away from it, within the metamerical limits of the

body. I have already mentioned it speaking of human metamerism in Chapter Four.

In the imaginative language we have used, we could say
that the somatic man suffers through syndromes of surface
pain and of deep somatic pain, the vegetative man suffers
through syndromes of visceral pain, and the two communicate
each other's sufferings in the form of referred pain.

So we have come to know a little better the nature of pain
and how complex it is. Health sciences have classified, analyzed, dissected the various aspects of pain from different view-
points, but have not yet been able to answer the central
question of the entire matter: Why is man suffering in the
dramatic way he does? Animals perceive the hurt, but they
do not suffer in the dramatic way we often do. Why are we
the only creatures on earth called upon to suffer? The answer
cannot come from medicine, but rather from religious philosophy. I submit that if man pays with diseases for his mistakes,
refusing to live up to his full human potential, in disease the
pain represents a kind of invitation to acknowledge the errors.
The suffering could almost be viewed as another key, along
with breathing, through which humans can in some way
arrange for the reunification of themselves.

If suffering can sometimes seem almost an insult to our
pride as technicians who have been able to put a man into
orbit and send him to the moon, it is unquestionable that
pain reduces the material man to humility. There is no difference between an emperor or a tycoon, and a thief or a beggar,
when they are struck by hepatic colic. Their suffering has
stripped them of their false glitters, and has taken them,
naked in their human reality, before the physician or the
priest. If their personality is well adjusted, there will be dignity and strength even in the deepest of pains. But if under
the false mundane glitters there was emptiness, the entire
personality collapses under the influence of pain, reducing
the human being to a ghost of his former self.

The balancing effects of pain and suffering have been
recognized since earlier cultures and civilizations. In primitive
societies, pain was identified with the "evil spirit," and as such
was exorcized through magic formulas, charms, and amulets.

Today we could call this set of magical practices the first attempt of psychotherapy to relieve pain through self- and hetero-suggestion.*

Historically, the notion of pain underwent a few transformations. From manifestation of an "evil spirit," it became the concrete expression of a punishment inflicted on man by some offended deity. Consequently, the means of treatment changed: no more magic formulas, but ritual sacrifices, prayers, and propitiatory ceremonies for the offended deity. Priests thus became the first physicians in the history of man: on their altars, they entreated the recovery of the faithful in exchange for offerings and cult sacrifices. This conception ruled medicine in Greek and Roman Ages, so much so that Hippocrates could write: *"Divinum opus est humanum sedare dolorem"* ("It is a divine task to soothe human pain").

With Christianity, the concept of pain underwent further modifications: It is no longer the manifestation of a divine vengeance, but a means of purification offered by God to man, to make him more submissive and sensitive to His Grace. In the Gospels, stories are frequent relating miraculous recoveries through devotion and faith in the Saviour Jesus Christ. These testimonies are all the more interesting when we recall that St. Luke the Evangelist was a physician and came from a school of Greek priest-physicians.

We may ask ourselves: Where do the recovery miracles narrated in the Gospels and in the stories of the saints of all religions mean to lead us? To a simple physical comfort? We have seen that there is no purely physical pain. The miraculous recovery from pain and from any other disease, in its deepest interpretation, is an invitation to man to return to himself, to heal the wound of his nature, to eliminate the errors of an existence too long lived against nature, to put him in harmony with the principles governing the Life of the Universe.

Historians have recorded diseases and physical tortures in the lives of many saints; but one thing is certain: the saint

---

* The english word "pain" stems from a sanskrit root *pu,* meaning "sacrifice." From the same root, the latin word *poena* (punishment) is also derived.

does not manifest the agonies of suffering in the same way we usually do. He endures his pain with peace of mind; in him, the enlightened Consciousness has been able to absorb the painful perception without triggering noisy pain complaints. His trained will power has been able to reject the painful physical sensation, transferring it to a higher level of spiritual acceptance.

Paramahansa Yogananda writes: "Sincerity, conviction, faith, deep intuition are like explosive bombs capable of making the mountains collapse. If these qualities were used to heal a disease, together with a strong Will, they can operate any desired change from evil into good."

Maybe at this point you will wonder: These are fine and very interesting words, but what use are they to us when we are in bed groaning from a fierce headache or from a paralyzing sciatica? Few of us can be "saints" to the extent of being able to sublimate our suffering. This is an unquestionable statement of fact, but it is not a human condemnation. I dare to assert that every man has the latent ability to prevent, limit, and, up to a certain point, control pain mentally through his will. How this is possible, I shall try to explain by following the thread of the techniques of self-control taught by Yoga.

In the first place, let's try to live in a healthier, more wholesome way: *yama, niyama*.

A great deal of visceral pain syndromes already find relief, and sometimes recovery, in the simple law of moderation. Let us eat less and better foods, and we will be able to control our stomach aches. Let us drink less, and our small liver ailments will disappear, our joint pains will come down to limits of possible endurance. Let us try to be well balanced and glad in every situation of our lives, noble in adversity, generous in abundance. Let us curb our material desires. Let us work wisely, without too much greed for profit, alternating work and proper periods of sound rest. Let us live as much as possible in the open air, away from the smoke of the cities, and we shall see our headaches disappear, our blood pressure become stable, our sight improve: we shall enjoy a new joy of living, totally unknown before. Let us curb our sexual overexuberance, using the genital activity according to Nature, and we shall see vanished our bladder ailments, our lumbar aches, our chronic tiredness that annoys us so much every morning, when instead we should and would like to get up from bed fresh, rested, happy for the new day which is starting. . . . Let us live in a natural way, and we shall suffer much less: a new energy will enter our life, rendering our work more constructive and our relationships with others more serene.

Some control over our habitual verbal complaints of pain should be included in the golden rules of moderation. Chronic bodily aches are a natural phenomenon, connected with the aging of our bony structures and internal organs, and should not be transformed into a drama to be played over and over again. Moreover, contemporary sociopsychological studies have shown that habitual pain verbalizations do not only reflect degrees of unpleasant perceptions, but also are the expression of cultural, familiar, and social patterns of emotional behavior.*

People from different cultures differ widely in their responses to painful perceptions. In connection with chronic back aches, an Italian is likely to be quite uninhibited, crying loudly to bring attention upon himself, whereas an Oriental probably will have a more phlegmatic, withdrawn attitude, with little moaning and groaning.

Consequently, the control of chronic pain complaints can be considered almost the first step toward achieving some inner freedom from the compulsion of habitual emotional outbursts. Ultimately, it could also be viewed as an aspect of *ahimsā*, an act of love toward our neighbor, whom we do not want to bother with endless descriptions of our ailments.

In addition to a well-balanced way of life, the body needs to be harmonious and nimble, in order to eliminate the "rust" of many years lived in an unhealthy way, to eject the toxins of hyperalimentation, violence, anger. The *āsanas* can eliminate muscular pains, pains from tension, syndromes from deep somatic pain. I don't need to repeat here what I have already mentioned in Chapter Four with regard to the therapeutical psychophysical effects of the *āsanas*. Instead I want to give an idea of some principles of pain therapy, so that

* Zborowsky M. *People in Pain* (San Francisco: Jossey-Bass Co., 1970).

afterward I may be able to compare them with similar effects obtainable through the *āsanas*.

Clinically, pain can be controlled along three main approaches: (1) by blocking the painful impulses at the level of the peripheral nerves—all the drugs with a local anesthetic effect, and drugs capable of reducing the spasm of the somatic and visceral muscles, work in this way; (2) by stopping the propagation of the painful impulses along the spinal cord—the so-called spinal anesthesias and some of the tranquilizing drugs operate in such ways; (3) by reducing the pain perception and reaction at the level of the brain centers, through drugs capable of dulling their function—sedatives and narcotics.

The action of all pain drugs is transitory, and present many habit-forming dangers that drive to progressively higher dosages, slowly raising the toxicity and diminishing the useful effect (just think of the very serious risk of drug addiction). We can assert that, more or less, every pain drug weighs negatively on the general economy of the organism, on the individual will, and on the energy patrimony (*see* Chapter Ten).

The *āsanas* act in some way along the same lines: (1) They eliminate a great many muscle spasms and their metameric referred visceral disorders; (2) they produce some beneficial effects upon the peripheral nerves entering the vertebral spine, through the movements of flexion, torsion, and extension of the vertebral column according to the various postures; (3) an excellent tranquilizing effect is achieved with the total body relaxation in *padmāsana* and similar relaxing postures; (4) finally, at the brain level, the pain perception is dulled and diverted by the mental concentration required for the correct execution of each single *āsana*.

Unlike the pain-killing drugs, the *āsanas* never affect the organism negatively. On the contrary, they energize the entire nervous system, help to control the sympathetic system, and ultimately enable the patient to reach a conscious self-control over the experience of pain.

I have already mentioned that pain, along with breathing, could be another key to restore man's unity, since his three separate parts make themselves loudly heard at the time of suffering. As a matter of fact, there are close relationships between pain perception and reaction to pain through the respiratory system. In the individual who suffers, breathing usually speeds up, becomes arhythmical, often dyspnoea appears. Also in common parlance, we assert the connections between pain and breathing when we say, "We have suffered pain which left us breathless."

In a man not trained to self-control, pain speeds up breathing. But this sentence can be reversed: being able to control breathing one can place pain under his conscious volitional control.

Again, we are back at the practice of *prāṇāyāma*. The control of breathing according to the technique of *prāṇāyāma* which has been mentioned in Chapter Five, allows for the conscious control of a pain syndrome through two possible methods: (1) a mental diversion similar to that obtainable with the *āsanas*: the mind, concentrated on the respiratory exercise, perceives the pain less intensely, consequently reducing its responses to it; thus, many collateral effects of pain on the heart, on the blood circulation, on the endocrine functions, are lessened; less cardiac arythming from pain, less blood pressure changes, less thyroid and suprarenal hormone unbalance; (2) through the conscious absorption of the *prāṇa* with breathing, the body is charged with vital energy that can be used to neutralize or to stop the painful impulses along the spinal cord. In other words, the Yogi learns to use the *prāṇa,* to close his spinal gate to most of the sensory inputs.

Let us try to explain this point further with an example. When you injure your hand or prick yourself, instinctively you clutch the injured part, squeezing it hard, almost trying to stop mechanically the propagation of pain to the brain. At the same time, you get excited and start hopping around. Behaving in this way, you unconsciously and confusedly execute a diverting maneuver, attempting to close your spinal gate. What you try to do at a subconscious level, the evolved Yogi does consciously, keeping a steady mental concentration on breathing and on his *Chakras*.

Only recently has medicine discovered the value of *āsana* and *prāṇāyāma* in controlling pain, and is applying them scientifically in what today is commonly called natural childbirth technique.

The pain from childbirth is not a natural phenomenon, it is not a necessary price to pay in order to bring a child into the world. In its innermost physiological mechanism, all the pain from childbirth should be limited to a sensation of compression on the uterus and of stretching on the muscles of the perineum. Animals deliver almost without painful manifestations and almost always without the least complication. In the woman, on the other hand, sometimes delivery is like a drama, with shooting pains declared unbearable, screams, sweatings, semifaints, multiple complications for the mother and for the fetus which is exposed for hours to the storm of a delivery that is no longer physiological.

About forty years ago, the English physician Richard Read had cleverly noticed that in the woman's pregnancy serious psychological factors of trouble and unbalance usually interfere: ancestral fears, domestic and tribal dreads and biases, emotional elements, conditioned by the way fecundation has occurred, gestation has taken place, the outside or inside "environment" formed around the central event, expected or feared at the end of the nine fatidic months. . . . These variable mental factors are unconsciously translated at the time of delivery into muscular tensions that act against what should be the neuromuscular and hormone mechanisms for a physiological expulsion of the fetus. As is well known, delivery occurs along three subsequent stages of muscular contraction and relaxation: autonomous tension of the muscles of the uterine body, auxiliary voluntary contraction of the diaphragm and of the muscles of the abdominal wall, relaxation of the neck of the uterus and of the perineum.

It is clear how an alteration in this sequence involves complications, delays, and pain. The parturient woman usually remains strained when she should relax in the intervening period of rest between two expulsive pushes. She spasmodically contracts her muscles, which she should relax; consequently she gets abnormally tired, and tends to relax just when she should actively cooperate with the automatic contraction of the uterine muscles during the expulsive stage of the fetus. The fetus clearly shows it is suffering from the alterations in the physiological sequence of expulsion, and sometimes it can pay for the psychological mistakes of the mother with its innocent life.

During the predelivery psychosomatic training, the pregnant woman is instructed to assume correct postures of muscular tensions and relaxations required by obstetrical physiology. At the same time, she undergoes a regular respiratory training to control the rhythm and the amplitude of her breathing consciously, in relation to the stages of muscular relaxation and contraction. With such training, she reaches delivery in psychophysical conditions similar to those characteristic of a Yogi. As soon as she feels the first stimuli to bear, she can assume the most suited physiological position to facilitate the subsequent stages in the expulsion of her baby. At the same time, she concentrates intensely on her breathing, so that the sensations of muscular contraction and stretching are perceived as such and no longer as pains from childbirth. The entire delivery work will go on consequently fast and regular, without screams, without dramas, with a child who will be born rosy and ready for his first joyful trill of greeting to life: his first act will once more be an "inspiration."

Chapter Nine

Yoga Concepts
Applied to
Contemporary Medicine:
Some promising
Attempts

It has only been a few years since contemporary medical science embarked on an extremely ambitious course, trying to apply a highly sophisticated technology to cure many diseases that only yesterday were considered hopeless.

Through progress in surgical, anesthesiological, endocrinological, pharmacological, bioengineering, and other techniques, medicine is attempting to attain recovery from every pathological lesion, from every medical or surgical disorder, even when delicate organs such as the heart and the brain are involved.

Specialized surgery would like to substitute worn-out organs and tissues with other organs obtained from human bodies deceased a short time before. Endocrinology is trying to use hormones manufactured in the laboratory, in substitution for the worn-out secretions of the endocrine glands. The pharmaceutical industry is producing an enormous amount of drugs, labeled useful to deal with all our mental probems—antianxiety and antidepressant drugs, tranquilizers and sedatives, stimulants and sleeping pills. Psychology is exploring the recesses of our brain correlates, trying to find the secret of their functions in order to correct and guide them. Neurosurgery would like to control all kinds of pains and aches by cutting or modifying the transmission and/or the reception of the sensory impulses. The ambition of the health sciences today is to make man, if not immortal, at least happy within prolonged limits of corporeal life.

Medicine is right in every attempt to deal realistically with human miseries as they are, but it is wrong in its ambition to solve problems of health and disease only from a corporeal standpoint. The health sciences will not be successful in their noble target to offer assistance and guidelines toward a happier life so long as they consider only the material well-being of the body, even through its psychological connections, and ignore the totality of the human being, made up of soul, mind, and body. Because of this basic mistake, most of the clinical attempts to go beyond a determinate therapeutical threshold have so far failed, or at least have partially deluded the promises born out of laboratory researches.

As long as physicians limit themselves to help natural processes in the healing work they may be successful. But when they want to take over Nature in order to heal, they meet invariably with a number of reactions of the organism, which seems to resist any trespassing against natural laws. Thus most of the attempts to transplant organs taken from a corpse have so far failed because of the prompt tissue defensive reaction that destroys and ejects the foreign organ as it were violating the biological intimacy of each individual.* All attempts to solve our daily wear and tear of life with drugs not only have failed but have produced tremendous problems of intoxication and addiction, ultimately resulting in our contemporary drug-dependent society. So also, many

---

* It is true that contemporary data show almost 80 percent success rate in transplanting kidneys, but this is achieved in an artificial way, depressing the defensive mechanisms of the body through life-long intake of corticosteroid drugs. Continuous depression of the bodily defenses dangerously exposes the patient to all kinds of infections from germs, to many endocrine and metabolic abnormalities, to a number of psychological maladjustments, of which transplant-medical centers around the world are becoming increasingly aware.

neurosurgical operations for the control of chronic pain by destroying nervous pathways, such as resection of nerve roots and/or resection of certain fibers in the spinal cord, have been disappointing on long-term evaluation of results, and often generated additional troubles, such as weakness of the limbs or several visceral disfunctions.

Even if surgery has been able to open a live and vital human heart, to lay bare a brain pulsating with life, too many times it has encountered human organisms that refuse to collaborate, in spite of every technical and electronic device, organisms which seem to thwart the cleverest maneuvers of experienced wizards of surgery. In surgery, the biological noncooperation has many names: surgical shock, painful scars and adhesions, multiple relapses, respiratory failures, and so on.

It is to be hoped that in the near future the health sciences will be able to combine our technological skill with a deeper understanding of the human wholeness, in order to provide a true and long-lasting help for our health problems. The key to health does not lie in drugs or surgical manipulation, but in an intimate, conscious adherence to the principles of right thinking and right living. The Yoga way of life, and any other serious spiritual discipline as well, are basically directed toward teaching the art of living, coming out of our miseries and diseases into a healthier and more joyous dimension of life.*

New ways of thinking are already evident among many intelligent and—perhaps—philosophically prepared health professionals. Silently, with caution, and almost a sense of fear, Western science is rediscovering the ancient wisdom and knowledge of the Orient, subjecting to experimental and clinical controls the truth discovered and manifested by the enlightened Masters of Vedic India. In the course of this

---

* The English words "right" and "righteousness" stem from a Sanskrit root *rita*. The same root appears in the word "ritual." In its semantic meaning, therefore, all rituals are nothing else but an invitation to righteousness and right living. Indeed, everyone who has ever deeply followed some beautiful rituals in churches of every denomination knows that for a while he felt great, as if he were lifted into a more joyous level of living experience.

book, some Western interpretations of Yoga training have been mentioned: physical therapy and rehabilitation, natural childbirth, Williams exercises (*see* Appendix).

The techniques of how to achieve control of our habits and how to overcome painful disabilities through voluntary efforts are certainly to be listed among the more advanced and daring Western interpretations of Yogic training, and should be briefly discussed here.

Operant Conditioning and the Control of Our Habits

In Chapter One, I mentioned that when an action is performed long enough, it becomes a habit, that is, a behavior that is learned both on the somatic and on the visceral level. We could define a habit as a mode of subconscious action shared by somatic man and vegetative man, often with the participation of endocrine man.

The American psychologist B. F. Skinner, in his well-known work *The Behavior of Organisms*, published in 1938, has distinguished two kinds of behavior, which he called "respondent" and "operant." A behavior is defined as respondent when it is under the direct control of a stimulus; it is defined as operant when it is controlled and reinforced by its consequences. A good example of these two different types of behavior is illustrated in the phenomenon of hunger versus appetite. Hunger is a peculiar feeling that is triggered by a visceral stimulus, reflecting the need for nutrition to preserve the life of the organism; appetite is a habit of taking pleasure from some kinds of food, being constantly sustained by the satisfaction of the organs of sight, smell, and taste.

Both respondent and operant behavior can be conditioned, that is, triggered without a specific act of volition; in the first case, the stimulus is always antecedent to the response, whereas an operant response is regulated by the events that follow it. Consequences that strengthen behavior are called reinforcers or rewards. In the example of appetite, sight, smell, and taste are reinforcers in conditioning food intake, independently of nutritional need, often against the patient's conscious will.

The distinction between stimulus-evoked behavior and operant behavior is not only academic, but has an important biopsychological significance. Living creatures are not merely machines responding to adequate inputs in simple, unchanged and stereotyped ways. They are intelligent beings responding to a variety of stimuli with a variety of learned and differentiated behaviors, which can be changed. We learn most of our habits during childhood and adolescence, when the learning processes are most active. Contemporary studies have shown that a great number of life patterns are preset since the early years of childhood, and are able to condition our behavior throughout our entire span of life. This fact emphasizes the tremendous importance of proper education during early stages of maturation. It also imposes a heavy responsibility upon parents and educators, who should be thoroughly trained to meet their duties in a comprehensive way, satisfying both the material, mental, and spiritual needs of young people. From Vedic India, the ideals of the *brahmachary* stage of education for young boys and girls seem to revive and offer assistance to the recent discoveries of Western social psychology.

In psychology, operant conditioning—or instrumental training—means those techniques that try to change behavior by acting upon and manipulating its consequences. Basically, these techniques first try to identify all reinforcers of any given behavior that must be changed. These reinforcers are then extinguished step by step, and are gradually substituted with other factors that are incompatible with the behavior to be changed. At the same time, these identical factors are directed to act as reinforcers for a new, proposed behavioral model. Thirdly, a variety of rewards is engineered in order to praise success along the way toward the proposed goal.

The field of clinical applications for the operant conditioning is wide and quite promising. Operant conditioning has been useful in controlling such habits as smoking, drinking, excessive appetite, and even some types of chronic pain, particularly where secondary gains—such as family attention or economic compensation—seem to reinforce the pain behavior.

Recently, several groups of scientists, from various university centers in New York, Baltimore, Boston, and elsewhere in the United States, have started a series of remarkably ingenious experiments, conducted with normal subjects and

patients, attempting to teach them how to control their vegetative functions. These investigators have used different operant conditioning techniques to teach subjects to change their
heartbeats, and to raise or lower their blood pressure. For
instance, in one experiment at the Massachusetts Mental
Health Center in Boston, volunteer students were trained to
raise or to lower the blood pressure: a flash of red light and
a simultaneous sound marked any change in blood pressure,
as recorded by a normal blood pressure cuff connected with
an electronic audio-amplifier. Success in raising or lowering
the blood pressure was rewarded by projecting on the screen,
after every 20 flashes, *Playboy* nude slides. The subjects were
instructed that the slides offered them an incentive to make
the red light flash as often as possible.*

The positive results of the study indicate that blood pressure can be modified by the use of external and operant
reinforcement. Studies are now under way in the same
Center to apply these techniques to the treatment of patients
who are suffering from high blood pressure.

In another health center in California, two leading scientists have worked with heart patients, and in a few cases have
slowed cardiac arhythmias from a range of 120 to 140 beats
per minute to a range of 60 to 70 beats per minute. In
periodic check-ups, these patients have shown some ability
to retain this learned control over pulse rate. In a third university center in the State of Washington, a team of psychologists and physicians is training patients with chronic back
pathology to increase their performances, *despite their back
pain*, using operant conditioning methods.

The implications of such research and observations are far-
reaching, even if it is too early to evaluate results in terms
of statistical significance. Evidence of learning in the vegetative functions removes the compulsive assumption that we
are a fixed product of evolution, enslaved to the automatic
working of vital organs, beyond voluntary control. Evidence
shows that our heart, our liver, our kidney, all our internal
systems, do not function like robots, but are conditioned to
factors that can be modified through learning. Ultimately,

* Report from *Roche Medical Commentary*, February, 1970.

we will find that health, as well as sickness, is a habit to be learned and properly controlled. Diseases do not usually come by accident, but are the consequences of wrong habits, as it has been repeatedly mentioned in the course of this book; they are also influenced by subtle cosmic forces, totally escaping our awareness, as I've already mentioned in Chapter Seven speaking of "Circadian Rhythms."

We are back to Yoya. In some ways, Yogic training could be considered the most ancient, and probably the most comprehensive, operant conditioning technique in the history of mankind. Its approach to a man is holistic: diet, physical and mental exercises, work, and rest, all receive due attention.

Using the language of psychology, we could consider *yama* as the identification and the extinction of wrong habits; *niyama* as the gradual construction of new, positive, behavioral models. *Āsanas, prāṇāyāma,* and other higher Yogic techniques train us for better levels of health and performance. The rewards will be experienced all along the path of training as ever-increasing feelings of peace of mind, intellectual illumination, joy and love, until—in *samādhi*—the Supreme Reward is achieved, realizing within ourselves our own Creator in a relationship of infinite Love and Joy.

There is, however, a profound difference between Yogic operant conditioning and its counterpart in Western psychology. This latter is an engineering artefact, an external manipulation from a source—the therapist—outside the patient. External manipulations do affect our inner functioning but this does not change the basic issue: individual will power. The only will power required of the subject undergoing psychological conditioning is to stay in the program long enough to achieve results. Everything else is left to the professional skill and motivations of the therapist; thus the results can never be better than the therapist himself.

On the contrary, in the Yoga discipline, the key point of success is the effort-making will power of the individual. The spiritual teacher gives the technique, but the disciple must make the effort on his own, removed from any outside manipulation. The Yogic methods are taught, but the experiences must be lived from the inside of the individual; in Western operant conditioning, on the contrary, the technique is not taught, but administered, and the experiences are preset by the therapist.

The Control of Psychosomatic Disabilities

Our daily lives are made up of various sequences and combinations of efforts. To "live" and to "survive" requires countless efforts of adjustment, understanding, compromising, overcoming, or accepting.

Basically, medicine classifies efforts in four main groups: (a) *Performing efforts,* like walking, talking, working, driving a car, and so on; (b) *Bracing efforts,* like standing or sitting erect —efforts by which we hold the body, or part of it, still and rigid; (c) *Attention efforts,* which enable us to understand events in our external environment or within ourselves (d) *Ideation efforts,* by which we can represent objects or events that are not actually impinging on our sense organs; thinking, remembering, anticipating, worrying, are examples of ideation efforts.

A well-balanced human being should be able to control and to coordinate all efforts, so that the total sum of his energy expenditures might be harmonious and goal-oriented. The more universal and spiritual these goals are, the higher the reward will be during our earthly journey and certainly in the Hereafter. However, most of us are poor managers of our energy expenditures. We are seldom capable of efficient effort-making, more often wasting our energies in useless and unrealistic targets of secondary importance. Moreover, because our organs and systems learn patterns of behavior, once any given pattern has been learned, it will be played again and again, compounding the possible effort-mistakes, until they are changed.

An example may be useful to illustrate this concept. Suppose we hurt ourselves: We will make some quick bracing and performance efforts in order to escape and prevent further hurt, while our blood pressure and our heart rate are likely to go up. The next time we anticipate a hurt, for instance sitting in a dentist's office, we unconsciously repeat the same bracing efforts, holding rigid throughout the dental procedure, with our blood pressure and heart beats soaring. The end result will be much more discomfort from back and other muscular tensions than the actual pain inflicted by the dental work; many faintings and collapses in the doctor's office have this learned origin.

Up to a certain point, mistakes in effort-making are common to all human beings, and do not generate serious disabilities. However, the effects of inappropriate efforts upon the nervous system, when excessive and above a certain, individual critical point, may give rise to a variety of so-called psychosomatic disorders, such as anxiety and depression syndromes, digestive system disturbances, elevated blood pressure, impotence and frigidity, headaches and back aches, chronic fatigue states, various obsessions and compulsions. Probably 75 percent of the patients waiting in the offices of general practitioners around the world belong to the class of poor effort-makers, otherwise identified as chronic sufferers and complainers. These unfortunate persons are usually making rounds from one doctor to the other, gulping down enormous quantities and varieties of drugs. Some of them undergo repeated and useless surgery. Others may be directed toward hypnosis or psychotherapy. None of these procedures seems to help them. As a matter of fact, they cannot. Drugs, surgery, hypnosis, are not likely to be effective, because they cannot teach a chronic sufferer how to perform better; no pill can teach a person how to drive a car or how to repair the water pipes in his home.

Only recently has medicine learned to identify and to regroup the different psychosomatic disabilities, otherwise scattered throughout all medical books, into a comprehensive and unitarian conceptual and clinical entity—the so-called "dysponesis." The word stems from the Greek *dys*—meaning "fault," "wrong"—and *ponos*—meaning "effort, work, energy."* Medicine has also learned very recently to provide alternative ways, other than drugs and surgeries, to deal effectively with dysponesis.

The general principles of management could be briefly outlined as follows: (a) to "desensitize" the patient to some particular sensory experience, in instances where he is prone to misdirect his efforts; in the previous example, the patient who

* Report on "Dysponesis," from *Behavioral Science,* vol. 13(2), March 1968.

has learned to be rigid in a dental chair can be trained to relax his useless bracing efforts by giving him some other performance task; (b) to provide him with some basic understanding of his disability, eventually teaching him to be aware of the maladjusted efforts he makes subconsciously; (c) to instruct him how to perform correctly some elementary bracing and performance efforts with minimal energy expenditure; (d) to bring him to differentiate discomfort from effort, and effort from emotions, so that he can gradually learn how to channel his emotions and perform better in any given situation; (e) to teach him step by step to observe and to judge himself in all his energy expenditures, and to watch, discriminatively, his performance.

We are back again to Yoga. I submit that Yoga is probably the most effective way to deal with various psychosomatic disabilities along the same, time-honored, lines of treatment that contemporary medicine has just rediscovered and tested. The *Āsanas* are probably the best tool to disrupt any learned pattern of wrong muscular efforts. *Prāṇāyāma* and *pratyāhāra* are extremely efficient techniques to divert the individual's attention from the objects of the outer environment, to increase every person's energy potentials and "interiorize" them, to achieve control of one's inner functioning. Moreover, in restoring human unity, the Yoga discipline is always increasing awareness and understanding of ourselves, adjusting our emotions, expanding our intellect, and enabling us not only to function better in any given situation, but to perform as spiritual beings with universal values.

Chapter Ten

Drugs,
Hypnosis,
and
Yoga

We have seen in the course of this book how contemporary medicine has come close to Yoga at various points dealing with our physical and mental functions. In this last chapter, I think it is useful to present some other points where Yoga and medicine are far apart in thinking. I'm referring here to drugs and hypnosis as ways to solve non-acute problems of pain and of other psychosomatic tensions.

Drug Problems

The use of narcotics and sedatives, derived from plant life such as poppy and mandragora, is perhaps one of the oldest forms of pharmacotherapy known to man. Early records, such as the Egyptian Ebers Papyrus and the poems of Homer, contain a few statements concerning the use of drugs to relieve acute pain from wounds. During the Middle Ages, a so-called *spongia soporifera* ("sleeping sponge") was a common sea-sponge soaked in a liquid mixture of poppy and mandragora juices. Its use must have been quite impredictable and hazardous, often resulting in permanent pain relief because of death. Historians have recorded several cases of patients undergoing amputations of limbs fully awake, rather than accepting the dubious and dangerous sleep from the "magic" sponge.

Historians agree that the use of pain-killing drugs was limited to acute and emergency situations. Once these were over, the drug intake was promptly discontinued. It is true that cases of drug abuse and addiction are as old as mankind, but it is also true that the abusers were considered outlaws and cast out of their communities.

Things have changed today. First of all, modern pharmaceutical industry has made the use of all drugs easier, safer, and more reliable. Secondly, our Western culture has become much more sensitive to pain and discomforts than our fathers have ever been. Nobody today would ever imagine enduring any kind of surgery, even minor surgery, without proper analgesia, as Western women more and more tend to deliver their babies without the least discomfort. Thirdly, the medical profession is relabeling as "medical problems" a number of "wear-and-tear" situations common to all humans, which only yesterday were viewed as simple, even if unpleasant, attributes of everyday living. This new mentality is well depicted in much well-known radio-TV advertising. For instance, in one of them it sounds something like this: "If you don't fall asleep within a few minutes after you have gone to bed, why wait? Take the sleeping pill X and sleep, sleep peacefully." The idea is introduced here that the pill *solves the problem of sleep,* totally overlooking the fact that sleep is a natural phenomenon, born out of physiological processes. Lack of sleep, therefore, is an indication that there are inner tensions and disharmonies in our body and mind, manifesting themselves through poor sleeping habits of which we are not aware. The drug intake may mask the problem for a little while, inducing an artificial sleep, but in the long run it surely makes it worse through habituation, drug dependency, and addiction.

The fact is that we have become a drug-oriented society. We have been conditioned to believe that drugs can solve all our daily problems, that medicine and the pharmaceutical industry have an answer to all questions of health and disease. We are instructed to take a pill in the morning in order to speed up our activities; a number of pills in the afternoon to quiet us down, to help our stomach digest our meaty and spicy meals; one or two pills at bedtime to help us to sleep peacefully. There is a little story among health professionals, illustrating this mentality: A patient goes to the doctor and is asked how does he feel. The answer: "I don't know, doc, I have not yet seen the report from yesterday's lab tests."

In order to discuss the position of the Yoga discipline toward excessive and unnecessary drug intakes, I want to mention briefly the mode of action in the best-known depressant drugs in common practice today.

1. *Opiates.* Under this generic name are found most narcotic drugs, including the well-known morphine and methadon. The site of action of the opiates is not well established. As shown in Diagram E 5, Chapter Eight, the narcotic-opiates probably slow down the emotional responses to painful and unpleasant sensations, acting upon some brain areas where the "bells ring" following sensory stimulations. There is also evidence that opiates depress the function of the vegetative nervous system, as shown by many symptoms of neurovegetative irritability during the period of withdrawal from narcotic addiction. In the usual imaginative representation of medical data, we could call the symptoms from narcotic withdrawal the protest of our vegetative man who was taught by his somatic twin to love the drug too much.

2. *Barbiturates.* Under this label is a large number of well-known sleeping pills, including "red devils," the street nickname for seconal, which is a barbiturate. Barbiturates are considered general depressants of the entire nervous system; as such, they are likely to smooth down both sensory inputs and motor outputs. Mental processes of evaluation, volition, and cognition are also reduced. The damaging effects of the barbiturates upon the whole nervous system are dramatically revealed in those generalized, life-threatening convulsions and seizures during the period of withdrawal from addiction. It is not only the vegetative man who protests here; all three parts of our disturbed individuality are affected by drug deprivation.

3. *Tranquilizers.* Under this name are labeled various groups of drugs sharing the common capability of slowing

down some of our nervous activities while inducing a mild muscular relaxation. The site of action and the addicting potentials of each tranquilizing drug are dependent upon its pharmacological structure, different from group to group. Most dangerous are those tranquilizers with a chemical structure very close to that of barbiturates. In these cases, the mode of action, the risk of addiction, and the withdrawal symptoms are almost identical to those of barbiturates.

In summary, we can safely state that the use of every depressant drug, no matter what its precise mode of action is, further reduces that little island of consciousness with which we identify ourselves. While this reduction of mental functioning is acceptable and may be useful in acute medical emergencies, it becomes extremely dangerous when chronically maintained.

Medicine is fully aware of the dangers connected with drug abuse, but sometimes it becomes trapped when the abuse is connected with chronic pain. The phenomenon of chronic pain —I mentioned in Chapter Eight—is often the expression of a disturbed personality, unable to cope with itself and with the environment. Pain, therefore, becomes almost an outlet for emotional discharges, having lost a great deal of its original meaning of "ringing the bell" in the face of a body damage.

Let me take an example. Suppose you have a chronic back ache from postural defects of the vertebral spine. You keep going so far as you are motivated to do so, despite your aches. But if one day your motivations to function go down, your back pain will become an unconscious way out of your duties. You therefore will channel through it all your frustrations. But your increasing complaints, *truly perceived and not faked,* sooner or later will bring you to medical attention and to a prescription of some pain-killer. If this pain-killer is a depressant drug, be it an opiate, a barbiturate, or a barbiturate-type tranquilizer, then your island of consciousness will start to shrink. The less you will be able to cope with your life, the more your conflicts will increase and manifest themselves in the form of additional pain. But more pain requires more drugs, with more mental confusion, and so on, until our little island of intelligence is flooded in the darkness of drug addiction.

There is increasing evidence among investigators at the University of Washington in Seattle that chronic pain behaviors are a socially acceptable way to seek drugs, not to cope with pain so much as with interpersonal life problems. The same investigators have recorded numerous cases of drug addiction for chronic pain in which dramatic improvements of mental and physical functioning were gained after taking the chronic sufferer off the drug.*

One explanation for the observed improvements is that the mental functions of the patient were expanded again following the drug withdrawal. Such expansion of the little island of consciousness first enabled the individual to recognize his interpersonal problems as such and no longer as pain. He then learns alternative and positive ways to deal with them in an operant-conditioning program of psychosomatic rehabilitation.

We come again to Yoga. Depressant drugs and Yoga are exactly the opposite: The former shrink consciousness, the latter expands it. Drugs lead to a progressive lowering and eventual annihilation of personality. Yoga drives man up to higher integrated states of consciousness ultimately translated into more harmonious human expressions.

I submit that Yoga training is one of the most effective techniques of operant conditioning to deal with problems of chronic pain, illness, and drug habituation. The teaching of modern Yoga does not go against the use of drugs to deal with emergency situations. While offering alternative ways to cope with emergencies, Yoga is realistic and acknowledges that the average disciple at our present stage of evolution is unlikely to develop high enough mental powers to *overcome all acute stress situations*. However, its teachings are a continuous warning against all drug intake. The right attitude should be to use the least amount of drug in order to get over the peak of any given pathological problem. Then one should quickly discontinue the drug and use *āsanas* and *prāṇāyāma* to take over, and prevent—or break—vicious circles of pain and sickness (*see* Diagram E, Chapter Eight).

* Quoted from Brena, Halpern, and Holcomb, *Pain Behaviors as Drug-Seeking Behaviors"* (in progress).

Speaking about drugs, I feel compelled to discuss here the question of the so-called "drug mysticism."

Health science has become interested in those pseudomystical experiences resulting from hallucinating drugs such as LSD. Words such as "super-consciousness," "illumination," "transcendental experience," have come out of the languages of the mystics and have entered the scientific laboratories. However, similarities of language and semantic expressions must not confuse the basic issue: LSD and other hallucinogenic drugs have a depressant action, however poorly understood, and probably limited to the sympathetic system.

The so-called "expansion of consciousness" experienced during an LSD trip is illusion. Our personality seems to go out of itself, whereas actually it shrinks below itself. The beauty of the trip, the awesome experiences described by some LSD users, only reflects their own pre-experiences as well-balanced personalities. The bad trips reported by others are the sad reflection of an unbalanced ego. This observation is further evidenced by the lack of observable improvement or change in the overall behaviors of LSD users following their trips.

In Chapter Two, I pointed out that the real value of every Yogic and other mystical experience is not too much what is said about them, but how they are translated into unselfish, universal services to others. No such behavioral standard of judgment can be applied to the "drug pseudomysticism," no personality improvement has been demonstrated following pseudomystical experiences. They are actually nothing more than another trap of our drug-oriented present-day mentality. As we want to escape our daily problems with sleeping pills and tranquilizers rather than solving them intelligently; as we want to escape the consequences of our sexual activities preventing with a tablet or killing that natural outcome designed by the species; as we are conditioned by our technology to expect everything in return for no personal efforts, so also we expect to find God with the help of a pill.

In the usual figurative language of this book, the LSD experience can well be compared to an abnormal overexpansion of the somatic man over his depressed vegetative twin. The predominance of the somato-sensory system over the visceral systems has been discussed throughout this book as one root cause of our disharmonies. The expansion of the somatic man following LSD intake consequently further disrupts the harmony among ourselves. It is everything else, but not *YO-GA,* that is, "Re-Union" through conscious, voluntary effort.

Drug pseudomysticism has, however, some deep positive aspects of which we are barely aware today. First of all, it helps to make the health scientist aware that there is something above and beyond our habitual states of consciousness. It has taken the metaphysical side of the human nature out of the vague, semitrue standards of occultism and has brought it into the light of open scientific investigation. In due time, health science will discover that spiritual training is not a matter concerning only saints and swamis, but a very practical aid to everyone's physical and mental hygiene. Science may disclose and test those treasures for healthy and happy living hidden in the teaching of Yoga and Zen, the "Spiritual Exercises" of St. Ignatius of Loyola, of St. Theresa of Avila, and of other great reformers of men.

Secondly, drug pseudomysticism actually masks a profound longing for God in our Western culture. As many of us take a depressant drug in an attempt to escape the solution of troublesome interpersonal problems, so others take LSD and other drugs of the same kind in an attempt to reach the desired goal—God—without making the proper efforts. It is possible and realistic to hope that many of those who have had a glimpse of the glorious reality behind our five senses during a "lucky trip" might be induced by the memory of it to seek more mature and constructive ways to reach in Self-Realization the knowledge of a Truth only dreamed of during the trip. Finally, the pseudomystic experiences recorded in connection with hallucinating drugs are helping to bring together, along with other factors, the health sciences and some organized religious institutions.

Constructive attempts toward establishing a common language between medicine and religion may work for a better integrated mental and physical hygiene in contemporary society.*

---

* For further information about Yoga and drugs, the reader is referred to a recent Yoga statement on the use of drugs, issued by the Self-Realization Fellowship, *Self-Realization Magazine,* 1970, Vol. 41/3.

Hypnosis

Like many other human thoughts buried by the centuries under heavy covers of misinterpretation and magic, hypnosis has come out only recently into the light of open discussion and scientific investigation. Actually, hypnosis is as old as man himself since it is a natural gift of the human mind which can be used either for healing or for less noble purposes. The movement from which modern medical hypnosis developed was inaugurated toward the end of the eighteenth century through the life-long work of an Austrian physician, Franz Anton Mesmer.

Mesmer had a deep intuition of the *prāṇa* as a universal all pervading force. He employed the term "magnetism" to indicate the relationship between cosmic forces in nature and man. He presented a physical theory according to which a "universal fluid" (*prāṇa?*) permeates the nervous system of living organisms as well as all other objects of creation. Mesmer elaborated upon his ideas and eventually came to the conclusion that many diseases are produced by a distorted "turn over" of the cosmic magnetism, disrupting the harmonious flow of the universal fluid in and out of man. He consequently thought that by concentration and manipulation of the magnetic fluid some diseases could be healed.

I do not know if Mesmer ever knew about the teaching of the *Vedas*,* but his concept of "magnetism" as a cosmic force interrelating with human lives is very close to the core of the Hindu ideas of *karma (see* Diagram C). Mesmer tested his ideas dealing with the practice of medicine, and was able to achieve through his "magnetic cures" some positive results in the management of a number of sick patients.

Mesmer's cures aroused sensational attention in Vienna, but also aroused cool and hostile reactions from the organized medical associations of his time. Passionate and dogmatic

---

* The *Upanishads* were translated from Sanskrit into European languages and introduced in Europe toward the second part of the eighteenth century. The thinking of some philosophers around the same period of time have close points of resemblance with Hindu thought. For instance, beside Mesmer and Schopenhauer, the "way to moral perfection"—of which Benjamin Franklin speaks in his *Autobiography*—has close points of similarity with the Yogic golden rules of *yama* and *niyama*.

attacks against hypnosis, criticisms, accusations of "black magic" and "witchcraft" went on throughout the nineteenth century, alternating with honest attempts at objective investigation and evaluation of Mesmer's ideas and "cures," then known under the name "Mesmerism." At the beginning of the twentieth century, however, there were fewer people still opposing Mesmerism on a religious or medical basis. By the second decade of this century, questions were no longer raised about the therapeutical potentiality of hypnosis in the management of some mental and physical disorders. Whereas its place in religion might still be disputed, there is no doubt that medical hypnosis is a well-documented technique, open to research and study.

Let us now briefly see what hypnosis is in order that we might discuss it in relationship with the Yoga way of thinking.

Hypnosis is a state of consciousness similar to being half-awake and half-asleep. It is induced through a single-pointed concentration of one's attention, while the surrounding areas of possible distraction are lowered until they are out of awareness. A simple example of this process can be found in the so-called "highway hypnosis" where the road's white line stretching in front of the driver acts as a "one-point concentration," while all the surrounding grounds are shut out of the driver's awareness. Once induced, hypnosis produces the following results: (1) an increased concentration of the mind: (2) a deep body relaxation; (3) a high susceptibility to suggestion.

By the simple definition of hypnosis, we can at once identify some points of contact with basic Yogic training, such as the profound body relaxation and the altered state of consciousness, one-point focused. However, the similarity ends here. The hypnotic state of consciousness is not an actual expansion of the mind-power through planned and coordinated training, but the result of an external manipulation of the therapist. It is true that the hypnotic concentration can be directed toward God and enable the subject to get a closer glimpse of eternal Truth. However—as Bryan has pointed out—this glimpse is an emotional experience that might be a little deeper than the formal church teaching on an intellectual basis, but far from that mystical "realization" of Truth, which is neither emotional nor intellectual, but purely intuitive, with a tremendous sense of certainty. States of Super-Consciousness always translate themselves into moral elevation, intellectual illumination, and other experiences that have already been discussed in Chapter Two. None of these have been recorded following hypnosis. Finally, the hypnotic state places the person in a position of dependence upon the therapist because of an increased susceptibility to suggestion. This situation may be useful to feed the patient with positive thinking, aimed at correcting a given health problem. However, there is little doubt that it restricts the moral freedom of the subject being hypnotized, who is actually giving it up to the therapist.

It has been said that many so-called "miracles" of instantaneous healing recorded in the Holy Scriptures of the world have been achieved through hypnotic suggestions. I am not debating this point. The wisdom of the sages and of the saints is not a matter that should be of concern to us. It is well possible that some "miraculous" healing was actually achieved through a hypnotic process. Saints and sages have their own ways to serve the suffering people of the world, and I am the least capable to discuss them. The point I'm trying to make concerns the fact that hypnosis is an external manipulation by a therapist, which does not require a personal, prolonged effort, nor a spiritual commitment. It does not generate an expansion of consciousness but rather a state of semisleepiness. It does not free the individual into a moral elevation, but places him in a relationship of dependence upon the therapist, not necessarily based on mutual love. In other words, hypnosis is not Yoga and should not be confused with any true mystical experience.

We could repeat here, in reference with hypnosis, what I have already said concerning drug pseudomysticism. There is no question that hypnosis is a useful medical tool. In some difficult medical problems of chronic illness it offers numerous advantages over drug therapies because of no known dangers of addiction. Hypnosis is and should become more and more a useful tool of research in the field of metapsychology. It reminds the health professionals that "there is something" behind our senses over and above the little island of consciousness we possess. At this hypothetical point of convergence health sciences and mystical teaching may soon meet.

Epilogue

In the course of this book, similarities between Yoga and medicine have been put in perspective and discussed in their relationship with different aspects of human phenomena.

We may ask ourselves: Besides more or less close similarities is there a realistic ground upon which both contemporary science and Yoga philosophy are going to meet and possibly to cooperate? The actual field of convergence between them lies in the recognition that physical laws of matter are binding men only to a certain point; beyond them, man can find inner freedom, using his will power and proper techniques to select his habits and to gain control of his visceral and emotional functioning, according to the principles of learning. Psychology tells us that our biological functions are bound to the rhythmicity of earthly phenomena, but it also has demonstrated that our performances can be controlled by instrumental training, which is not influenced by circadian rhythms. It looks as though scientific investigations from one side are showing man bound to the earth, like any other living creature, while from another side they seem to prove that the human potentials are greater than the forces binding us—which is exactly what the

Vedas have been teaching for thousands of years. The concept
of "dysponesis" is much more than a new theory in medicine.
It is almost a new philosophy, bringing into perspective the
value of energy-spending in problems of health and disease.
Because of our habitual lack of control over our visceral systems, we are often too prodigal in spending our energy capital.
In any given situation, we are not only prone to "overshoot,"
but also to learn the "overshooting" as a mode of habitual
interreaction with our environment. We are always tense and
aggressive in whatever task we perform, always in competition
with somebody or with ourselves, wasting our energies in confused actions and maladjusted reactions. We often do not cope
with some given situation following a rational and intelligent
evaluation, but with emotional outbursts, burning out a lot
of fuel. The experiences gained from the various rehabilitation
centers around the world, dealing with a variety of disabilities,
confirms that our potentialities are greater than we assume,
provided that we adequately train our energy-spending and
effort-making.

Operant conditioning and dysponesis management have
barely started to explore the ground of clinical applications.
They are now at a stage of development that can be compared
to surgery one century ago, a few years after anesthesia was
discovered in 1846. On the other hand, Yoga has been teaching for centuries that the secret of fulfillment in life and
spiritual evolution lies in the ability to concentrate vital energy
instead of dissipating it.

The "Royal Way of Yoga" takes man as he is, with all his
handicaps, and brings him above boundaries of material forces
to Cosmic Consciousness, teaching him how to expand his
energy capital and how to use it wisely. Along the way, while
he is seeking spiritual realization, man can also discover the
key to health, joy, and inner freedom.

In this field of thinking and teaching, the age-old Yoga discipline and the more advanced investigations in health sciences
have actually met and do agree.

In this Appendix are some visual representations of a few simple physical exercises commonly suggested in medical practice, which have points in common with the Yogic techniques.

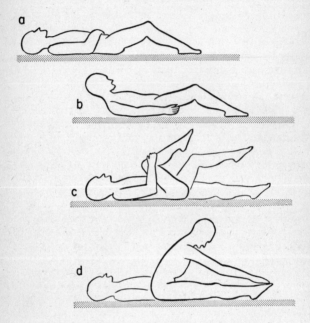

"Williams exercises" for postural correction

FIG. 8 presents four exercises for postural correction (the so-called "Williams exercises"). These exercises are designed in order to correct painful postural defects of the vertebral column due to wrong bracing habits and/or to pathological process of the vertebral articulations. Fig. 8a shows how to correct an abnormal curvature of the vertebral spine in the lumbar region by moderately bending the legs at the hip and the knee joints. Fig. 8b, c, d reproduce the basic principles of the *āsanas*, with positions calling for rhythmical contractions of various groups of antagonistic muscles (flexors and extensors). The bending and the extending of the vertebral column ultimately lead to improved performance and decrease of subjective backache.

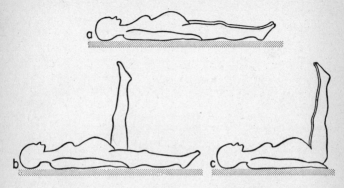

Fig. 9

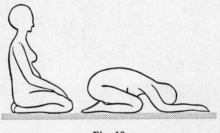

Fig. 10

Training for "natural childbirth"

FIGS. 9 and 10 present two exercises suggested in the training for "natural childbirth." Fig. 9a first shows a position for perfect relaxation, similar to the equivalent Yogic posture. In Figs. 9b, c again you can see points of contact among these postures and similar *āsanas,* while Fig. 10 is practically the same as the *Yogamudra* (Fig. 7).

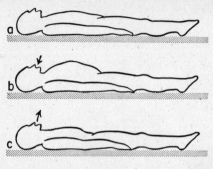

Fig. 11

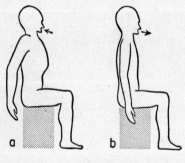

Fig. 12

Basic breathing exercises

FIGS. 11 and 12 show some basic breathing exercises. Exercise 11a again shows a position of perfect relaxation. Exercise 11b shows the correct way to inhale, first using the diaphragm, then the chest muscles. Exercise 11c shows the correct way to exhale, reversing the movements of b. Exercise 12 repeats the same respiratory movements and emphasizes in 12b the relaxation achieved through a period of expiratory apnoea, while keeping the spine straight and erect.

The illustrations are intended as examples, and by no means should be attempted without medical supervision.

Physical exercises look like the equivalent Yogic techniques, but should not be confused with them. They do not teach how to control the vital energy within ourselves, and do not consistently influence mind activities. Yoga, on the contrary, uses physical training in order to achieve and control, first, and then to expand, the mind power, using the vital energy aroused through the physical training. In other words, Yoga is not a medical technique, while it has much to offer to medicine. It is a *spiritual training* to be taught and practiced under wise spiritual counseling through qualified Yogic Institutes.

References

1   Arnold, E., *The Song Celestial: The Bhagavad Gita.* London: Routledge & Kegan.

2   _____ *The Light of Asia: The Life and Teaching of Gautama Buddha.* London: Routledge & Kegan.

3   Bryan, W. J., *Religious Aspects of Hypnosis.* Springfield: Thomas.

4   Bucke, R. M., *Cosmic Consciousness,* 25th edition. New York: Dutton & Co.

5   Chatterji, M. M., *The Bhagavad Gita.* New York: Julian Press.

6   Dutt, R. C., *The Ramayana & The Mahabharata: Notes and Selections.* New York: Dutton & Co., Everyman's Library.

7   Evans-Wentz, W. Y., *Tibetan Yoga and Secret Doctrines.* London: Oxford University Press.

8   _____ *The Tibetan Book of the Dead.* London: Oxford University Press.

9   Gandhi, M. K., *A Gandhian Rosary: Selections from the Teaching of Gandhi.* Ahmenabad, India: Nabajivan Publishing House.

10 _____ *Autobiographie: Mes Experiences de Vérité.* Paris: Presse Universitaire de France.

11 Herbert, J., *Krishna, dieu d'amour.* Paris: Albin Michel.

12 Legge, J., *Texts of Taoism.* New York: Julian Press.

13 Lewis, M. W., *Life Story.* Los Angeles, Calif.: Self-Realization Fellowship.

14 Mishra, R. S., *The Textbook of Yoga Psychology*. New York: Julian Press.

15 Mouni, S., *Ways to Self-Realization*. New York: Julian Press.

16 Muzumdar, S., *Yogic Exercises*. Bombay, India: Orient Longmans.

17 Radhakrishnan, S., *Eastern Religions and Western Thought*. London: Oxford University Press.

18 _____ *The Hindu View of Life*. London: Allen & Unvin Ltd.

19 _____ *The Brahma Sutra: The Philosophy of Spiritual Life*. New York: Greenwood Press.

20 Riley, F. E., *The Bible of the Bibles: A Source Book of Religions*. Santa Barbara, Calif.: Rowny Press.

21 Skinner, B. F., *The Behavior of Organisms*. New York: Appleton.

22 Spalding, B. T., *Life and Teaching of the Masters of the Far East*. Los Angeles, Calif.: De-Vorss & Co.

23 Tagore, R., *Toward University Man*. New York: Asia Publishing House.

24 Teilhard de Chardin, *The Phenomenon of Man*. New York: Harper.

25 Vivekananda, S., *What Religion Is*. New York: Julian Press.

26 Yogananda, P., *Autobiography of a Yogi*. Los Angeles, Calif.: Self-Realization Fellowship.

27 _____ *Science of Religion*. Los Angeles, Calif.: Self-Realization Fellowship.

28 _____ *Scientific Healing Affirmations*. Los Angeles, Calif.: Self-Realization Fellowship.

29 Yohnson, C., *The Yoga Sutra of Patanjali*. London: Watkins Co.

30 Yukteswar, S. S., *The Holy Science*. Ranchi (Bihar), India: Yogoda Satsanga Society of India.

31 Ministry of Education, India, *Report of the Committee on Evaluation of Therapeutical Claims of Yogic Practices*.

32 *Self-Realization Magazine*. Los Angeles, Calif.: Self-Realization Fellowship.